# THE NEW RULES OF LIFTING SUPERCHARGED

# THE NEW RULES OF LIFTING SUPERCHARGED

## Ten All-New Programs for Men and Women

**Lou Schuler** and
**Alwyn Cosgrove**

**AVERY**
A MEMBER OF PENGUIN GROUP (USA) INC.
NEW YORK

Published by the Penguin Group

Penguin Group (USA) Inc., 375 Hudson Street, New York, New York 10014, USA · Penguin Group
(Canada), 90 Eglinton Avenue East, Suite 700, Toronto, Ontario M4P 2Y3, Canada (a division of Pearson
Penguin Canada Inc.) · Penguin Books Ltd, 80 Strand, London WC2R 0RL, England · Penguin Ireland,
25 St Stephen's Green, Dublin 2, Ireland (a division of Penguin Books Ltd) · Penguin Group (Australia),
707 Collins Street, Melbourne, Victoria 3008, Australia (a division of Pearson Australia Group Pty Ltd) ·
Penguin Books India Pvt Ltd, 11 Community Centre, Panchsheel Park, New Delhi–110 017, India ·
Penguin Group (NZ), 67 Apollo Drive, Rosedale, Auckland 0632, New Zealand (a division of Pearson
New Zealand Ltd) · Penguin Books (South Africa), Rosebank Office Park, 181 Jan Smuts Avenue,
Parktown North 2193, South Africa · Penguin China, B7 Jiaming Center, 27 East Third Ring
Road North, Chaoyang District, Beijing 100020, China

Penguin Books Ltd, Registered Offices: 80 Strand, London WC2R 0RL, England

Most Avery books are available at special quantity discounts for bulk purchase for
sales promotions, premiums, fund-raising, and educational needs. Special books or
book excerpts also can be created to fit specific needs. For details, write Penguin
Group (USA) Inc. Special Markets, 375 Hudson Street, New York, NY 10014.

Library of Congress Cataloging-in-Publication Data

Schuler, Lou.
The new rules of lifting supercharged : ten all-new muscle-building programs for men and women / Lou
Schuler and Alwyn Cosgrove. —Revised edition.
pages  cm
ISBN 978-1-58333-465-2 (hardback)
1. Weight lifting.   2. Muscle strength.   3. Physical fitness.   I. Cosgrove, Alwyn.   I. Title.
GV546.3.S39        2012                          2012039859
796.41—dc23

Printed in the United States of America
1  3  5  7  9  10  8  6  4  2

BOOK DESIGN BY TANYA MAIBORODA

# Acknowledgments

FIRST THANKS GO TO MY COAUTHOR, Alwyn Cosgrove, whose ten training programs are the main reason this book exists. His creative solutions to the problems we all face never cease to amaze me. The rest of our team has done the typically outstanding work we've come to depend on to make each New Rules of Lifting book better than it otherwise would be: Megan Newman and Gigi Campo at Avery; photographer Michael Tedesco and his assistants, Danelle Manthey and Matt Minor; Dan Ownes and Alli McKee, our ridiculously strong, knowledgeable, and cheerful models; Mike Cerimele, Chris Leavy, Brian Zarbatany, and the rest of the staff at Velocity Sports Performance and Steel Fitness Premier in Allentown, Pennsylvania, who are so generous with their time, equipment, and facilities for our photo shoots; and David Black, Gary Morris, and the rest of the staff at the David Black Agency.

As a journalist who struggles to understand the complexities of exercise and nutrition science, I'm utterly dependent on and grateful to the experts who share their research and knowledge with someone who barely got through high school math and chemistry:

- Brad Schoenfeld and Bret Contreras (exercise science)
- Alan Aragon and Mike Roussell (nutrition)
- Mike Nelson (current research)
- Stuart Phillips and Rob Newton (who not only shared but also patiently explained their own studies to me)
- Lonnie Lowery and Joey Antonio (all things protein)
- Jon Fass and Shon Grosse (physical therapy)

Alwyn and I could write the greatest workout books in the history of Western literature, and no one would ever find out if it weren't for the help of our friends in the media, who let potential readers know that our books, however much they fall short of the "greatest" standard, can help them reach their goals. Thanks to Adam Campbell, Nick Bromberg, Sean Hyson, Adam Bornstein, Pete Williams, Scott Quill, Jimmy Moore, Andrew Heffernan, Nate Green, and countless others who have helped us over the years. Thanks also to Jason Lengstorf and his Web design crew at CopterLabs.com.

Once again, I'm grateful to my friends Roland Denzel and Chris Bathke for reviewing early chapters and offering valuable feedback (none of which included "find another career," although with some of the earliest drafts it might've been tempting to suggest). Same goes for Otto and Aoife Hammersmith, who design the free NROL training logs at werkit.com.

I couldn't do this without the support I receive from my wife, Kimberly Heinrichs, and our three children, who graciously wait until I'm off deadline to pretend they need parental guidance.

I want to dedicate *The New Rules of Lifting Supercharged* to all my friends at jpfitness.com, including of course Jean-Paul Francoeur and, less obviously, John Gesselberty, whose grumpy enthusiasm for training inspires me. The friendship and respect I share with the JP Fitness community is the payoff for the paradox of long, sedentary hours at my desk to help others become more healthy and fit.

—L.S.


I want to take this opportunity to thank all of you, the loyal NROL readers and followers, for supporting us five times over.

Lou Schuler: Thank you once again for continuing to believe in me and my ideas about fitness training. Thanks as usual to Adam Campbell, along with all the lecturers, coaches, authors, colleagues, and seminar hosts I've learned from over the years. As I've said before, my growth begins with your willingness to teach.

To Chris Poirier and the Perform Better team, thanks for the opportunity to share what we do at Results Fitness with trainers around the world. To Lee Burton, Michael Boyle, Gray Cook, Todd Durkin, Jason Ferruggia, Jim Wendler, Craig Ballantyne, and Mark Verstegen and the Athletes Performance team: Thank you all for the inspiration to improve each and every day.

Robert Dos Remedios, you're a friend and a solid professional. I've learned so much from you. Thanks too for not hiring me all those years ago. It worked out well for both of us.

To Derek Campbell, my tae kwon do instructor and original mentor, and still the greatest coaching mind I've been fortunate enough to learn under. I've said many times that you changed the direction of my life, and I won't stop saying that I have no idea where I would be were it not for you. I'm forever grateful for the life lessons you taught me. The entire coaching world should be studying you, so hurry up and get your book written.

To Craig Rasmussen and Mike Wunsch: You continue to put the "pro" in programming. To my family at Results Fitness: Thank you for changing the way fitness is done. And to the Results Fitness University members: Keep up the great work.

To Terry McCormack, my very first weight-training partner: Thanks for the encouragement, support, and friendship over the years. Sorry about the prowler flu that time. And to Kerry McCormack, the most inspirational human being I've ever met: My universe will never be the same.

To Darren Vella: There's never a quiet night when we're hanging out together (and I remember them all). Thanks for each one.

To team 164, Mum, Dad, and Derek: I hope I've made you proud.

To God, and in no small part to Dr. Sven De Vos and the elite team of doctors and nurses at UCLA who saved my life and gave me these extra days here. I don't know why I deserve these days, but I'll never take them for granted and will always treat them as a gift. If it weren't for you, this book wouldn't exist.

And as always to Rachel, my soul mate and business and life partner: You say it best when you say nothing at all.

—A.C.

# Contents

**PART 3**

## THE SYSTEM

**PART 4**

## THE PROGRAMS

**PART 5**

## THE POSTGAME

# THE NEW RULES OF LIFTING SUPERCHARGED

# Introduction: NROL 5.0

IN THE BEGINNING, ALWYN COSGROVE AND I wrote a book called *The New Rules of Lifting*. And it was good. Readers liked it, and they got outstanding results from Alwyn's training programs. You wouldn't be reading the fifth book in the series if the first one hadn't helped lifters like you reach your goals.

But here's the thing: Most lifters like you haven't heard of Alwyn, or me, or the NROL series. Millions of men and women lift weights, either at home or in commercial gyms, but it's hard to see much evidence to suggest they're getting what they want from it, or what they could get from it.

Instead, I see all the same behaviors and practices that inspired us to launch the series in the first place.

I see paunchy middle-aged men block the dumbbell rack as they grind through set after set of every biceps exercise they remember from *Flex* magazine circa 1995, while avoiding the exercises that use the body's biggest muscles in coordinated action, the movements that would do the most to build muscle, burn fat, and turn back the clock to the days when they looked more like a page from *Men's Health* than *Cigar Aficionado.*

I see apparently healthy women doing the beneficial exercises the men avoid—the squats, deadlifts, and rows—but with weights that wouldn't challenge someone twice their age, with half their strength.

I see young lifters doing exercises that will turn them into old lifters, the moves most likely to cause injury and least likely to offer much benefit. I see older lifters doing half-baked versions of programs designed for young athletes or bodybuilders, only without any apparent sense of the mechanisms that would make such a program work.

It's like they've all gotten the first half of the memo about the importance of strength training for health, fitness, and appearance. But somehow the rest of the memo—the part that explains what you need to do to get the results you want—got deleted. So, in a way, the NROL series is the second half of that memo.

Take the first New Rule of Lifting: "The best muscle-building exercises are the ones that use your muscles the way they're designed to work."

Or the third: "To build size, you must build strength."

Or the twenty-third: "Results come from hard work."

Or the forty-third: "You can't protect your spine by doing exercises that damage it."

Or the sixty-third: "You're not a kid anymore. Don't train like one."

See what I mean?

The readers who found and implemented the original *New Rules of Lifting* (along with the ones who read *NROL for Women, for Abs,* and *for Life*) know what it means to *train*. They know how to lift in a way that allows them to get progressively stronger, to add more muscle, to reduce fat, to work *with* their bodies rather than *against* them. They're the ones who walk past the machines in their health club and pick up free weights. They're the ones who get stronger over time, at any age, despite roadblocks or limitations. They're the ones who look like they know what they're doing. They move with purpose. They sweat, they grimace, and every now and then they actually grunt.

Does that describe you?

If so, great. You're either a satisfied NROL reader, coming back for the newest information and most up-to-date programs, or you're a target reader, someone who's ready to do what it takes to get leaner, stronger, and more athletic.

Not you? Pull up a chair, and let's talk.

# THE POWER OF PROCESS

Since this is the Introduction, I should introduce myself. I'm a journalist who's been writing about exercise, nutrition, and weight loss since 1992, when I was hired as an editor at *Men's Fitness* (a magazine I hadn't heard of until I interviewed for a job there).

I met Alwyn seven years later, when I was fitness editor at *Men's Health* magazine and he was a personal trainer at a gym in New York City. He had been training clients since 1989, and working at it full-time since 1995, following a successful career as a competitive martial artist in his native Scotland. Alwyn and his wife, Rachel, opened Results Fitness in Santa Clarita, California, in 2000. They've logged every workout for every client since then, as well as the outcomes. Their database, which today includes tens of thousands of workouts, shows them what works to make their clients bigger, leaner, stronger, and in many cases healthier over time.

By the time Alwyn and I started writing *The New Rules of Lifting* in 2004, we had both been around long enough to know what we didn't want to do. We didn't want to write yet another workout book filled with before-and-after photos of people who'd gotten extraordinary results from Alwyn's programs. He had plenty to show, but we both understood the perils of promising outcomes to readers who didn't fully understand the process that leads to success in the weight room. We decided instead to focus on that process.

Our first goal was to show readers how a trainer like Alwyn puts programs together. Whereas a typical man or woman will view their muscles as parts of a machine that can be reshaped into more aesthetically pleasing parts—make *this* more dramatically contoured, make *that* less embarrassingly pockmarked—Alwyn looks at a client's body as an integrated system. Can he do basic movements pain-free? Can she stabilize her lower back and engage the right muscles in the correct sequence when lifting something heavy off the floor?

The second goal was to give readers a realistic way to achieve the outcomes everyone wants from strength training. For that Alwyn created ten programs, based on the ones he used successfully at Results Fitness. We showed readers multiple ways to sequence the programs to create a customized, yearlong training system. And, like I said, it was good.

Mostly.

Almost from the beginning, we found ourselves answering the same questions from readers.

First, there was the gender issue. While there's nothing in the original book that requires a Y chromosome, it never occurred to me that women would want to do Alwyn's programs. At the time the book came out—early 2006—you just didn't see women deadlifting, squatting, or attempting to do chin-ups. I didn't realize that a lot of them wanted to, and there wasn't anything in print that gave them an NROL-type plan to learn the lifts and use them productively.

The solution to that problem was obvious enough: We wrote *NROL for Women,* which came out in early 2008. We couldn't have asked for a more enthusiastic response from readers, which continues to this day. If that had been the only problem we had with our first book, we could've stopped right there.

But it wasn't.

The second problem, you could say, was evolutionary. Alwyn created the original *NROL* workouts in 2004, and the *NROL for Women* workouts in 2006. His methods have changed in both large and small ways since then, but the first two books still reflect exercises and techniques that he no longer uses with his clients.

We wrote *NROL for Abs* to address mobility and core strength, two keys to successful training that we'd underplayed in our early books. We followed that with *NROL for Life,* which addressed perhaps the biggest source of questions from readers: "If I can't do this exercise, is it okay to do another exercise instead? If so, which one?"

Eventually, all the new books brought us back to where we started. If we were writing *The New Rules of Lifting* today, with the same ambitions to emphasize the process of training and show readers how to custom-build a workout system, how would we do it?

## TRUTH IN LABELING

*Supercharged,* like the original *NROL,* includes ten workouts. The first four, which we call Basic Training, do everything you'd want a solid workout system to do: They give you time to develop or improve your exercise technique. They help you build, rebuild, or improve your overall base of muscular fitness, including strength, endurance, and joint mobility. Inexperienced lifters will develop at least a little muscle everywhere, and some male lifters will build a lot. Even experienced lifters will see improvements, especially in areas they've neglected. And everyone will burn lots of calories. So if you have fat to lose (and honestly, who doesn't?), you'll lose some of it with these programs.

You may wonder why an experienced lifter would do the same program as a novice, and it's a fair question. The truth is, it's *not* the same program in practice. The seasoned lifter is using more advanced exercises (which I'll explain in detail in Part 3), and he or she employs a level of force production that isn't available to the newbie. Well-trained muscles, put into action with well-honed technique, can lift more weight, lift that weight more times, and tap deeper into the body's energy reserves. The workout design may be simpler than a longtime lifter is used to, but that's a benefit. The more swipes we put on our gym-membership cards, and the more complex our workouts get, the farther we move away from basic exercises and techniques. We lose what we don't use, as the poet said, and thousands of *NROL* readers can attest to the benefits of returning to basics, even for a short time. (Full-circle training is an important theme in *Supercharged*, and one of the most valuable lessons I've learned from my many years of working with Alwyn.)

Basic Training I, II, III, and IV are followed by Hypertrophy I, II, and III. The workouts are similar to those in *NROL*, employing a system called undulating periodization to make muscles bigger and stronger. You'll vary load (working with heavy, medium, and light weights on different days) and volume (more total sets and reps when you're using lighter weights, less when you go heavier).

The final three programs are called Strength & Power I, II, and III. Pure strength is often the one component of muscular fitness that lifters neglect, even experienced ones. That's why a lot of readers of *NROL* and *NROL for Women* found that the programs requiring them to lift the most challenging weights produced the most surprising results.

## THE IMPORTANT STUFF

Here's what else you get in *Supercharged*.

In Part 1, I'll describe the basic movement patterns you need to master to be a successful lifter, and to successfully change the way your body looks and performs:

*Squat* (bending at the knees and hips, as you would before a jump)

*Hinge* (bending at the hips to lift something from the floor)

*Push* (pushing yourself off the floor, or pushing a weight away from your body)

*Pull* (pulling yourself up to something, or pulling something toward you)

*Lunge* (lifting with your legs in a split stance and both feet on the floor)

*Single-leg stance* (variations on the squat, hinge, and lunge movements in which only one foot is on the floor)

Then we'll look at the qualities you need to perform those movement patterns safely, effectively, and productively:

*Stability* through your shoulders, spine, and pelvis

*Mobility* in your hips, upper back, and shoulders

*Balance* that allows you to work in a variety of positions and postures

*Strength,* which is the ability to generate force

*Power,* which is the ability to generate force at maximum speed

*Endurance,* or conditioning, which is the ability to repeat all these movements, separately or in combination, often and vigorously enough to give your body the stimulus it needs to build strength, add muscle, and strip fat.

Part 2 gets into the physiology of muscles. What makes them bigger and stronger? The answer to the first question can be perfectly simple: lift progressively heavier things on a regular schedule, give your muscles enough food to grow, and give your body time to recover. The longer you lift, however, the more complex it gets.

Part 3 lists the exercises, followed by the workouts in Part 4. The ten training programs are the heart of the book. But you can't use them to your best advantage until you understand how to choose the best exercises for you in each part of the program.

Part 5 wraps things up with the questions many of you will want to ask. How do I know what you'll ask? Well, it *is* the fifth book in the series.

## WHO IS THIS BOOK FOR?

Alwyn and I write every book with the readers of our previous work in mind. We want to share with you the newest findings from the world of strength and conditioning research, as well as the closest approximation possible of the workout programs Alwyn and his trainers use at Results Fitness. Since Alwyn's team constantly updates their methodology, there's always something new to share.

If you're among the millions of experienced lifters who never heard of Alwyn, me, or the NROL series until you picked up *Supercharged*, I first want to thank you for giving us a shot. I also want to warn you that your first exposure to Alwyn's workouts can be mildly confusing. You'll be underwhelmed when you look at them on paper, and wonder how it could possibly be enough work to achieve your goals. Please trust me on this: It's plenty of work. You'll know from the first workout that these programs are uniquely challenging, and by the last workout you'll know they deliver as well as advertised (if not better). Please read carefully to ensure you get the best possible results from the system.

If you're an inexperienced lifter, or someone who's contemplating that first foray into the free-weight area of your health club after months or years of wasting your time on the machines, we're asking you to give our system a fair shot. I think Alwyn's workouts are an ideal system to get what you want from strength training. Are they the best? I have no way to know, because I haven't tried everything, and research can never quantify the infinite ways to mix and match exercises and techniques. This is as close as I can get to a definitive statement: Any plan is better than no plan, and going from machine to machine just because that's the way your gym chose to arrange its equipment is *not* a plan.

Conversely, there are some readers who will probably be disappointed.

If you're a competitive athlete in a strength and power sport, *Supercharged* can put you on the right track. But to reach your full potential, you really should seek out a specialized program specific to your needs. Alwyn has trained athletes in just about every sport, and he competed in tae kwon do at the international level. If he were writing a program for his younger self, or for a college or professional athlete, he would start with a template similar to the ones in *Supercharged*. But the application would be unique to that athlete and his or her sport. In addition, there'd be more of just about everything. We start every NROL book with the idea that our readers are willing to train about an hour a day, three days a week, which is a fraction of the time great athletes devote to strength and conditioning.

Which brings me to another type of lifter who might not like *Supercharged*: If you want to work out five or six times a week, or enjoy training for a couple hours a day, this probably isn't the right program for you. It's certainly not a traditional bodybuilding program. We don't believe in grinding through set after set of exercises designed to target the body's smallest muscles. Nor do we believe in using machines in which you move a bar or handle along a fixed path. The exercises in *Supercharged* will hit your biggest, strongest muscles using a barbell, dumbbells, kettlebells, bands or cables, or your own body weight. They take some balance and coordination. Your smaller muscles still get lots of work, but it'll come in support of the prime movers, which continues a theme we've emphasized throughout the NROL series.

The final category of lifter who won't like *Supercharged* is the one who is, to put it delicately, intractable. This is the guy who's been doing things his own damned way since high school, or the woman who remains so mortally afraid of "bulking up" that she avoids weights a preteen girl wouldn't hesitate to lift. (You'll see what I mean in Chapter 10.) They might understand the need to do something different, even if it involves a learning curve or a perceptual shift. But they'll use every excuse in the world to avoid a novel system that might make them feel momentarily awkward or uncomfortable.

Our goal isn't to make you feel threatened, since fear is a condition that prevents new ideas from taking root. We understand that this might not be the right program for you at this moment. If you change your mind, we'll always be here. Wait long enough and there'll probably be another NROL program for you to try. We never stop learning new ways to reach our goals, and we can only hope that you'll come to appreciate the many ways we've found to help you reach yours.

# PART 1

# WELCOME TO THE CLUB

# Membership Has Its Drawbacks

THE ADS CHASE ME across the Internet. It doesn't matter if I'm on a news site, a sports site, a political site, or a place that offers nothing more than a chance to waste time. (Which, come to think of it, describes many of the news, sports, and political sites I visit.) Wherever I am, Internet sites have me pegged as a musclehead, but not a particularly bright one. They think I'll be so intrigued by "This 1 trick adds 50 pounds of muscle!" or "5 foods you should never eat!" or "57-year-old mom looks 25!" that I'll stop what I'm doing, click on the link, and give some infomarketers my money, in hopes of becoming as buff as the model in the Photoshopped stock image they used to get my attention.

Make no mistake: I would *love* to have a secret formula to produce any or all of those magical outcomes. I'd put it in a book, sell millions of copies, and then write another book about how to write a book that sells millions of copies. But, alas, I know there's no single trick for building muscle, no foods that melt fat, and no product—animal, vegetable, or chemical—that will make any person in midlife look as young as a grad student.

I know those things don't exist because I have the burden of knowledge, a burden that Alwyn and I are about to impose on you. Not secret knowledge, like a roadmap to the lost continent of Atlantis (which, my sources tell me, wasn't a continent so much as a really nice vacation resort), or the key to wealth and fame (pretty sure it doesn't include writing books about strength training), or even one simple trick to get the physique you've always wanted (unless "pick different parents" counts as a simple trick).

No, this knowledge is out there for anyone to find. It tells you how to train in a way that produces the results you want over an unspecified amount of time, typically six to twelve months, provided you're willing to put in focused, consistent effort.

The information only appears to be secret when you consider how few of our fellow lifters seek it out and apply it. About 21 percent of American adults lift at least twice a week. But look around your local gym. (If you work out at home, find a nearby gym and stare through the window.) How many people are doing the most fundamental exercises—squats, deadlifts, presses, pulls—with good form? Let's make it even easier: How many people are even *attempting* the first two exercises—squats and deadlifts—with any kind of form, good or bad?

You, however, will do better. Why? Because you know the New Rules of Lifting, v. 5.0.

## NEW RULE #1 • It's great to be good.

You've heard the joke about how success is mostly about showing up. It's not true, as you'd know if you ever showed up for a job you hadn't been hired to perform. (Not saying I have, just that I'm pretty sure it wouldn't work.) Showing up at a gym, or in the room at home where you keep your weights, doesn't make you a lifter.

Self-efficacy is one of the biggest roadblocks to a successful workout program. People who believe they can follow through on a commitment to exercise will, in turn, exercise more often. Interestingly, they'll also tend to believe they can improve their diet, which leads to better eating habits.

Just believing you can do something isn't proof that you can do it well; history is filled with examples of tragic overconfidence. But it's the best starting point you can possibly have. As a study in the *Journal of Strength and Conditioning Research* noted, "Individuals' levels of motivation are more directly tied to what they believe to be true, rather than to what is objectively true."

Belief that we're good at something starts with one or more of these events:

- *A mastery experience*—that is, knowing that you've done something well.
- *A vicarious experience*, meaning that you saw someone like you do something, and came to believe you could do it.
- *A social-persuasion experience*, meaning that someone whose opinion you trust convinced you that you can do something.
- *Your physiological state* at the time you attempt the task; some days we just feel stronger or weaker, and that affects our confidence.

Of those, mastery is the most powerful indicator of self-efficacy, and self-efficacy is the best predictor of effort. The more confidence you have in your ability, the harder you will try. The harder you try, the better your results will be.

Alwyn and I don't want you to be confident because you *think* you know how to lift. We want you to know how to lift. That's why the first goal of *Supercharged* is to help you become a good lifter by learning the most important movement patterns, practicing them, moving on to more advanced variations of those movements, and using them to change the way your body performs.

## NEW RULE #2 • Once you're good, you need to get strong.

Out of curiosity, I Googled "why is strength important?" Almost every hit on the first few pages answered a question I didn't ask: "Why is strength *training* important?" If you care about muscular fitness, you know why it's important to train for it. Nobody reading a book called *The New Rules of Lifting* needs a litany of reasons to get your butt in the weight room and strategically relocate some iron while you're there. It's not broccoli. The goal of our hard work isn't to board that little black train a month or two later than we would have without the hard work. It's to feel better, look better, and do better *now*. Or at least soon.

But strength itself is often the last consideration of strength-training programs. Exercise is typically presented as a laundry list: "Do 3 sets of 10 repetitions of the following exercises . . ." Sometimes you see an admonition to use the most weight you can handle with good form. But even that seems increasingly rare. Fitness magazines—especially those for women—tell you to address specific concerns with specific exercises, rather than encouraging you to improve your performance in the exercises you already know how to do.

I'm a big fan of variety; my favorite workouts are the ones when I try something new. The more you learn, the more skill you acquire. That leads to confidence and self-efficacy. But new exercises, for all their benefits, won't lead to increased strength or muscle size unless you use them consistently and improve your performance in them over time. By then they're no longer "new." They're just exercises.

Learning a new exercise is a neural process. First your body coordinates your muscles and joints. Then it figures out how to use them efficiently. If you don't increase the weight, the exercise gets easier over time, which means you accomplish less with each subsequent workout. That's still better than not doing anything. Exercise burns calories, develops muscular endurance, and offers any number of metabolic and physiological benefits. But you don't have to settle for "at least I'm not on the couch."

The specific benefits of strength training come as much from the *strength* as the *training*. More strength means you can apply more force to each repetition. More force means more stress on your muscles, which produces three beneficial outcomes:

1. Your body uses more energy to perform the lifts.
2. Your body uses more energy during recovery.
3. Your body adds more tissue to the muscles themselves, a subject I'll return to many times in *Supercharged*.

That's why we work out.

## NEW RULE #3  •  "Strong" is an aspiration, not an endpoint.

Some of us are born with the potential to be much stronger than the average lifter in the average gym. Some of us—me, for example—take years to reach a point of general above-averageness, and take pride in our hard-won competence, the triumph of not accepting "Well, I totally suck at *this*" as the final answer. Maybe some of you reading this won't even hit average. Doesn't matter.

If *Supercharged* is your first serious lifting program, you may see tremendous strength increases in your first few months. You can easily double the amount of weight you use on exercises you're learning for the first time. But if you're an advanced lifter, you know that gains are hard to come by. A low-single-digit increase in strength over twelve months might be a breakthrough. A couple of pounds of new muscle, or maintaining the same amount of muscle while losing a bit of fat, is a nose-thumbing win against your genetic limitations.

It's all relative.

Your goal is to move forward: to get stronger, to get leaner, to develop more skill, to improve your athleticism, to get better at reading your own body so you know when it's safe to push harder and when your muscles and joints need a break. If you're the competitive type, make sure you compete against yourself, against the history of what your body can and can't do, rather than imagining that you have to rise to anyone else's standards.

## NEW RULE #4 ● The only *guaranteed* way to get strong is with a focused, progressive program.

As I write this, CrossFit is probably at the height of its popularity. It's a type of training in which each workout is an all-out effort, with the goal of making you better at all-out efforts. I can see the benefits for military and law enforcement personnel. No way the Will Smith character in *Men in Black* runs down an unlicensed cephalopod on foot without a next-level mix of strength, power, endurance, and fatigue resistance.

But a program based on wiping yourself out every time in the gym with a random mix of unrelated exercises will not help you reach your highest possible level of strength or muscular fitness. For that, you need a system that offers predictable challenges, set up so you improve your performance in incremental steps over a long period of time. Alwyn's *Supercharged* programs give you about ten months' worth of training—more if you decide to repeat some of them. That may or may not be enough time to reach your peak. If you're a novice, you're probably years away from hitting whatever ceiling your age, genes, and ambitions impose on you. An advanced lifter may hit personal records on all his lifts during Strength & Power III.

The only guarantee is that you won't ever know how strong or muscular you can get unless you focus on those goals for a year or more, making steady improvements in skill, strength, muscularity, and overall fitness. Skipping around from program to program, or from challenge to challenge within a system like CrossFit, is certainly better than not training at all. If it's the only way for you to enjoy lifting, by all means follow your bliss. Just understand that it's not the best way to reach your full potential as a lifter.

## NEW RULE #5 • To stay strong, you must move well.

This is really a multilevel concern:

1. If you have a lingering injury or imbalance, you can make things worse by adding more weight to your lifts.
2. If you don't have an injury, you sometimes create one by repeating the same movements over and over with increasing weight.
3. Either because of #1 or #2, many lifters adjust their lifting technique; shorten the range of motion; apply weight-room Band-Aids like belts, wraps, or straps; or (and this is probably the big one) shift to simpler, machine-based exercises because they allow them to lift more weight.

In every case, you make the same mistake: Instead of addressing a problem (something hurts or feels less comfortable), you exacerbate it. I tell you this because I've done everything I just described, and I see fellow lifters going down the same path.

You can head off a lot of problems with a dedicated warm-up routine, which Alwyn calls RAMP, for *R*ange of motion, *A*ctivation, and *M*ovement *P*reparation. It's followed by core training in the *Supercharged* programs. RAMP and core training should typically take fifteen minutes, plenty of time to get your muscles and joints thoroughly prepared to lift.

The second defense is the workout system itself. Without exception, I move better when I do Alwyn's programs as written, and worse when I veer off toward whatever I'm most interested in. I'll do my favorite exercises first, and avoid the ones I struggle with. Alwyn, thanks to his many years as an athlete, coach, and gym owner, knows which movements people like us try to avoid. He often puts them first in a routine, when you're primed to do them well. Those movements—the ones that make you feel awkward or uncoordinated—are often the ones our bodies need if we want to excel on the exercises we actually enjoy.

The third way to protect yourself is with skill—doing each repetition of each exercise with good form and the ideal range of motion.

Finally, there's recovery. Stretching and using a foam roller at the end of a workout is the first step toward preparing your body for the next workout.

## NEW RULE #6 • This means you.

As a journalist who specializes in exercise and nutrition, my job sometimes requires me to debunk whatever nonsense bubbles up at any given moment. One of the first I went up against was SuperSlow training, the idea that if you do excruciatingly slow repetitions on specially designed machines, you get all the benefits of traditional strength training in a fraction of the time. It couldn't possibly have been true, since it upended everything we know about how to get bigger and stronger. But it took years for research to prove that it didn't work as well as its supporters claimed, and in the meantime many believed that the inventors of SuperSlow really had found a loophole in the basic tenets of exercise science. (Some, I suppose, believe it to this day.)

And don't even get me started on the idiocy of "cleanses" and other enema-enhanced starvation diets that purport to remove built-up fecal matter and toxins that your body hasn't stored in the first place. It's an entire industry built from a single line in *Beverly Hills Cop*. ("You know, it says here that by the time the average American is fifty, he's got five pounds of undigested red meat in his bowels.") Bottom line, if it involves a body-penetrating rubber hose in a nonmedical setting, it's not a good idea.

The toughest arguments, though, concern good ideas that are carried too far. I wouldn't call SuperSlow a good idea, but everyone concedes that short, difficult workouts do *something*, and something is almost always better than nothing. They just don't do everything. This applies to yoga, Pilates, running, Spinning, martial arts, boot-camp classes, pole dancing, or anything else that claims to offer all you could ever want in a single exercise system.

You can't get strong without a program designed to develop strength. You can't build muscle unless you do the things that we know will force your muscles to get bigger. You can't make your body leaner unless you eat and train to accomplish that goal.

There really are no loopholes. Efficacy + strength + the desire to improve + a solid program = results.

Alwyn and I make no special claims for this particular program. There's no magical formula that Alwyn alchemized in his secret laboratory. Nothing here rewrites the bedrock principles of exercise science or defies the laws of thermodynamics. We believe in things that have been proven (gravity—that's a big one), and have no patience with things we know aren't true.

We like to think of ourselves as the guys you turn to when you give up on the idea of a quick, easy, simple solution to the problem of too much fat, too little muscle, or the dreaded combination of the two: skinny-fat. Our solution isn't quick. It isn't easy. Nor is it especially simple; it takes some concentration and patience to get the hang of it if you're new to the NROL series.

But it *is* a hell of a program—more detailed and sophisticated than any we've seen in print. That's as far as I'll go with marketing. Turn the page, and we'll get into the information you need for the results you want.

# The Six Movements You Need to Master

IN THE ORIGINAL *New Rules of Lifting*, we proposed that all exercises are based on six basic movements: squat, deadlift, lunge, push, pull, and twist. Locomotion—walking and running—represented a seventh movement category. We expanded on that in *NROL for Abs*, when we described three categories of core exercises. And then in *NROL for Life* we added a few more.

Lesson learned; there's no simple, indisputable way to classify exercises. But I think most veteran lifters can identify with this sentiment: If I could go back in time and talk to myself as a novice lifter, I would advise young, skinny Lou to master these six movement patterns: squat, hinge, pull, push, lunge, single-leg stance. The first four merit their own rules, and then I'll explain why Alwyn gives the other two their own categories.

## NEW RULE #7 • A real lifter knows how to squat.

A perfect squat is a rare and magnificent sight. Few lifters in commercial gyms attempt it, and only a small fraction of those do it well. "Perfect" will be slightly different for each lifter, but the basics remain the same. It starts with your hips moving backward. In the bottom position, the tops of your thighs are parallel to the floor, or slightly lower. Your center of gravity is over the middle of your feet, which are flat on the floor, and your torso and lower legs are leaning forward at more or less the same angle. Your toes are pointed out slightly.

Then you rise to the starting position along the same path you used to descend.

If you can squat with good form, you can probably do all the basic exercises well. It doesn't matter which variation we're talking about. It could be a goblet squat, in which you hold a weight against your chest. It could be a front squat, in which you hold a barbell across the front of your shoulders, or a back squat, in which you . . . well, you can guess where the barbell goes on a back squat.

They all require a combination of two qualities that a poor lifter won't have:

1. *Stability*, meaning you can brace the muscles responsible for keeping your body balanced as you descend and rise.
2. *Mobility*, meaning that your hip, knee, and ankle joints can operate smoothly and efficiently.

Mobility without stability leaves you unable to hold your back and pelvis in a safe, neutral position. Stability without mobility forces muscles and joints to work differently. Stiff ankles might shift more stress to your knees, while a deficit in hip mobility could put more stress on your lower back.

In *Athletic Body in Balance*, physical therapist Gray Cook lists the reasons why a squat can be difficult for an adult today. If you sit all day, there's a good chance that some of your muscles have gotten weaker, shorter, or tighter than they should be. An extremely active person who repeats the same movements for hours a week, like a runner, will also have muscles that have gotten shorter and tighter. The issues are different for the runner vs. the sitter, but both will have trouble squatting with good form and a full range of motion. Same with someone who's been injured. Scar tissue can form, limiting the range of motion in one area and forcing other parts of your body to compensate.

The beauty of the squat, done correctly, is that it helps you rewire all the muscles and movement patterns that have gone astray.

Start with the body-weight squat. If possible, stand sideways to a full-length mirror so you can assess your form. Set your feet shoulder-width apart, toes pointed forward (for now; you can turn them out slightly during your workouts). Hold your arms straight out in front of you. Push your hips back and lower your body until the tops of your thighs are parallel to the floor.

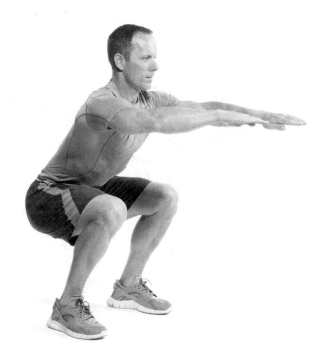

If you took a snapshot of yourself in this position, you should be able to draw a straight, vertical line from your shoulder to the middle of your foot. That's your center of gravity. When you squat with a barbell—no matter if it's on your front shoulders or your back—it should be directly over the same spot.

Now rise back to the starting position. You should be able to do this without moving your feet in or out. Moreover, you should be able to do this repeatedly, at least fifteen times without changing your form, before you're ready to squat with a weight.

## NEW RULE #8  •  A well-trained butt is a thing of beauty.

I attended a graduate writing program at the University of Southern California from 1991 to 1993. I got a lot out of it: my wife (we met and married in 1993), my career (I started at *Men's Fitness* magazine in 1992), some good friends, and an acute appreciation of my limitations as a writer (for a helpful overview, scan the one- and

## Eight Fun Facts About Squats

A 2012 review of squat studies in the *Journal of Strength and Conditioning Research* is a gold mine of information about the world's best exercise:

**1.** The front and back squats use two big lower-body muscle groups—the hamstrings and quadriceps—in the same way.

**2.** All else being equal, the more you lift on any squat variation, the more muscle you activate. That's why it's so important to increase your strength over time.

**3.** You can probably lift more weight on the back squat if you take a wider stance, and rotate your thighs outward. That increases activation of your glutes and adductors (inner-thigh muscles), but not your quadriceps and hamstrings, which are the prime movers.

**4.** Muscle activation is highest when your thighs are parallel to the floor. Cutting a squat short allows you to use more weight, but with less work for the muscles you're trying to build.

**5.** Going below parallel at the bottom of the movement increases activation of your glutes, but not your quads and hamstrings. Thus, you may get better overall muscle development with the front squat, since most of us can go deeper than we can on the back squat.

**6.** You activate 43 percent more muscle squatting with free weights vs. a Smith machine, the barbell on rails found in some good gyms and all bad ones. This is despite the fact that most people can lift significantly more weight on the Smith.

**7.** It's not just because you recruit more stabilizing muscles when you use free weights. The quads and hamstrings—along with the gastrocnemius, the main calf muscle—also work harder than they do on a Smith machine.

**8.** Same goes for the leg press and leg extension. Even though you can move a lot more weight on a leg press, nothing beats lifting a heavy weight on a vertical path with no help from a machine.

two-star reviews of my books on Amazon.com). To my surprise, I also gained a new understanding of gluteal-muscle activation.

One of the best young writers in the program was a Cuban-American woman who wrote a short story about how she learned to walk in a way that caused men to reject two million years of human evolution. The key, she wrote, was to give your gluteals a theme song as you walked: "For me, for you, for me, for you . . ."

For male readers, that translates to: "Shaka boom, shaka boom, shaka boom, shaka boom . . ."

So let's try a quick experiment. Get up from your chair (hard to activate muscles when you're sitting on them), and try the shaka-boom walk. Take a short step forward with your right leg (that's the "shaka" part), and finish the stride with a conscious glute contraction (the "boom"). Repeat with your left leg.

Looks weird, I know. Probably feels weird too; few of us are accustomed to conscious activation of our gluteal muscles, much less gratuitous activation. But if you can't get your glutes to fire on demand, you can't master a basic movement called hip extension, and if you can't master it, you can't perform deadlifts safely and effectively. That leaves you without one of the very best muscle-developing, strength-building, body-changing exercises ever invented.

In the traditional deadlift, you bend forward from the hips, lift a weight off the floor as you straighten your body, and then lower the weight back to the floor. You'll learn multiple variations on this movement in *Supercharged*. But they all require you to activate the prime movers, your glutes and hamstrings, while keeping your lower back and pelvis in a safe, neutral position.

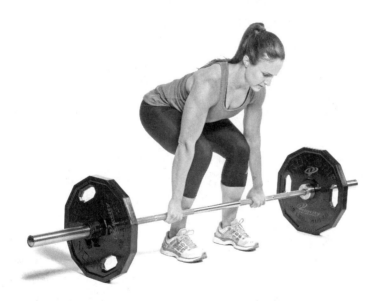

The original *NROL* used the word "deadlift" to describe the entire hip-extension category. In subsequent books, including this one, Alwyn classifies them as "hinge" movements. Visually, it's a perfect model for hip extension. Your hips act as a hinge as you bend your torso forward and then straighten it, powered by your glutes and hamstrings.

## What Is This Thing You Call "Training"?

I've used words like "exercise," "workout," and "training" many times already without explaining what I mean. To me, *exercise* is any purposeful movement that you do with the goal of improving or maintaining some aspect of your fitness. Shooting free throws or hitting balls at the driving range are exercise, in that you're working on skills that will make you better at basketball or golf. Going out for a run, or a hike, or a ride is also exercise. Conversely, something you do at a leisurely pace, like walking your dog, is physical activity, which is great. But it isn't really exercise; there's no performance-related goal beyond ensuring your dog doesn't pee on the carpet.

A *workout* is exercise that's deliberately strenuous, a stimulus that requires a period of recovery. You can exercise whenever you feel like it, but a workout is usually something you plan.

A *training session* is a workout with the goal of creating one or more specific biological adaptations—strength, hypertrophy, fat loss, speed, endurance, and/or skill.

You'll get the best results from the *Supercharged* workouts if you treat each one as a training session. But there will certainly be days when a good workout is the best you can hope for, and there's nothing wrong with that.

## NEW RULE #9:  •  Your lats are core muscles. Get off your rump and train them that way.

The latissimus dorsi—the wing-shaped muscles that sweep across the middle and sides of your back—take up more real estate than any other muscle group. They aren't the strongest muscles; your gluteus maximus holds that distinction. But they're probably the most versatile.

Their textbook role is to pull your upper arms to the sides of your torso. It's a huge assignment, crucial to climbing, rowing, swimming, or anything else in which you need to pull something toward you or pull yourself toward something. You'll do a pulling exercise in every *Supercharged* workout—some variation on the row, pulldown, or chin-up.

The *way* you do those exercises, however, will be different from what many of you expect.

To understand why, we need to look at the latissimus in detail.

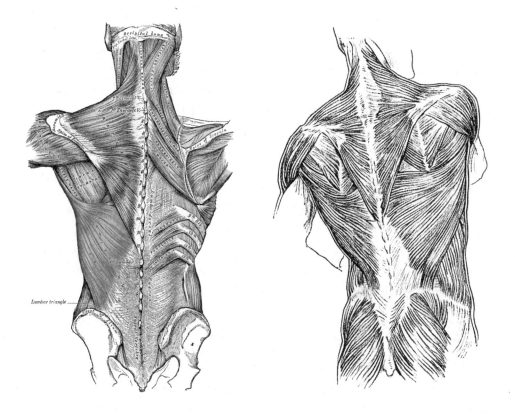

The muscles' fibers originate along the lower half of your spine, the top of your pelvis, and a big ol' sheet of connective tissue in between. That connective tissue, the lumbodorsal fascia, extends all the way to your tailbone. On the way down, it wraps around your erector spinae, the columns of muscle on either side of your spine.

That's how your lats become part of your core, which we define as the muscles that work to stabilize your spine and pelvis. They're the Kevin Bacon of musculoskeletal anatomy: a star in some movements (the pulling exercises), and a crucial supporting player in deadlifts and squats, in which they help safeguard your lower back. One way or another, the lats work with everything from your forearms to your glutes. Climbing, for example, employs a synchronized pull with one arm and hip extension with the gluteal muscles on the opposite side. Left arm, right glute. Right arm, left glute. In between the lat and glute, of course, is your lower back, which the lats are helping to protect even while they're engaged in a pulling movement.

Now consider the two most popular gym exercises that target the lats. There's the lat pulldown, in which you sit with your legs braced under a padded bar, and the seated row, in which you sit with your feet up on supports in front of you. What happens when you sit? You cut your body in half. You certainly use the lats to pull a bar toward your body. But by sitting on your butt you prevent that co-contraction with the glutes that provides stability for your lower back.

The lat pulldown and seated row share one other characteristic: They're typically done with god-awful form. Newbies will hunch their shoulders on the seated row, which prevents the targeted upper-back muscles from doing much of anything, while meatheads will do a limbo-like move on the lat pulldown, leaning so far back that they're using everything *but* their lats to move the weight.

That's why Alwyn's gym doesn't even have a station for doing seated rows. His clients do tons of rowing exercises, but they do them in positions that allow the lats to act as both a prime mover and a core stabilizer—standing, prone, hanging from a chin-up bar. They have a lat-pulldown station, but it doesn't have a seat. To use it, you have to either kneel or stand, forcing you, again, to stabilize your core while working your lats and the other upper-back muscles.

## NEW RULE #10 • Nobody ever died of small pecs.

There was a time when lifters didn't obsess over the size, shape, and strength of their pectoral muscles. It was before my time, but we aren't talking about ancient history. The bench press as we know it barely existed in the 1930s. Those who lifted focused on exercises in which the weight typically started on the floor and ended up overhead. At best, the bench press was considered an accessory exercise for the overhead press, which was part of Olympic weightlifting until 1972.

Before World War II, bodybuilding contests in the US were sanctioned by the Amateur Athletic Union, which also ran weightlifting. Sometimes the contests were held on the same day, in the same venue, with a few of the same guys competing in both. Some of the best bodybuilders were also good weightlifters, and some of the best weightlifters were also respectable bodybuilders.

America's best lifters were sponsored by York Barbell, and most of them trained together at the company's gym in Pennsylvania. York Barbell was owned by Bob Hoffman, who also published a magazine called *Strength & Health*.

Up in Montreal, a young guy named Joe Weider idolized Hoffman, and wanted more than anything to be just like his hero. Because Hoffman had a stranglehold on Olympic lifting, Weider needed a new niche. He focused on bodybuilding. Hoffman and his writers did all they could to disparage Weider, mocking his obsession with "pecs" and "lats," gay-baiting lifters who focused on looking good, and even accusing

Weider of pro-Communist sympathies. (I worked for Weider in the 1990s. *Not* a Communist.)

Weider had the zeitgeist on his side. The all-American energy and enthusiasm from the Muscle Beach scene launched a wave of interest in physique training in the 1940s and beyond. Olympic lifting ebbed in popularity in the 1950s just as the Soviet Union and its satellites started to use it as a propaganda tool. American weightlifting dominance ended in the 1960s, while the sport of powerlifting took off among those who wanted to be as strong as they looked. (Strange as it seems now, the biceps curl was originally part of powerlifting competition, along with the squat, bench press, and deadlift.)

To tell you the truth, I think Bob Hoffman had it right. The focus on physiques has certainly popularized strength training; it's why I have a career writing about it. But I don't think the focus on the barbell bench press, which Weider proclaimed "the king of upper-body exercises," has done any good.

I say that as someone who agrees with the basic rationale for the exercise. When I could do barbell bench presses with a somewhat heavy weight (by my own standards), I got bigger and stronger. I'm pretty sure I also damaged my shoulders, or at least set them up for injury. In retrospect, the craziest thing about my intermittent pursuit of a bigger bench is that it was never a comfortable exercise for me. It almost always made something feel worse.

And for what? What benefit could come from having a chest that's slightly bigger than it might've been had I stuck with a mix of push-ups and dumbbell presses? It's not a rhetorical question. When you look at classic sculpture from Greece and Rome, you see the physiques of young men who're lean and ripped. (The women are pretty hot too; Google "Roman sculpture Venus" to see what I mean. They don't look like lifters, but some of them suggest the models were in pretty good shape.) They look much more like the pre–bench press lifters and athletes at Muscle Beach than contemporary bodybuilders or powerlifters. Their waists are a bit thicker than today's standard, and their arms, chests, and lats aren't especially pronounced. But they still represent what would've been a muscular ideal for most of human history.

If you have no plans to compete in bodybuilding or powerlifting, I don't really see the point of bench pressing with a barbell. Alwyn rarely uses one with his clients and athletes, and as I've said, my aching shoulders wouldn't let me return to it even if I wanted to.

Instead, most of the emphasis in Alwyn's *Supercharged* programs is on the push-up. With the many variations shown in Chapter 10, many of you won't even need to advance to dumbbell presses until you get to the Hypertrophy and Strength & Power programs. Dumbbells work just fine with those programs, and your shoulders will probably thank you for choosing them over the barbell.

## LUNGE AND SINGLE-LEG STANCE

The lunge is as old as exercise itself. But until recently you rarely saw a guy use it in a workout program. Women, on the other hand, seemed to use lunges to the exclusion of the squats and deadlifts at the heart of programs written for men. Alwyn's an equal-opportunity coach: He wants both genders to work their butts off with the exercises that produce the biggest benefits for the time and effort you're willing to invest.

That the lunge is a crucial movement pattern is self-evident. Outside the gym, how many activities that require strength and power are performed with the feet parallel to each other and shoulder-width apart? Training your body to lunge in multiple directions, and from multiple heights or depths, will not only help your sports performance, it will do amazing things for your musculature. Readers often ask why we don't include specialized exercises for the calves, and every now and then someone will ask about training the inner- or outer-thigh muscles. Spend a few months doing Alwyn's workouts, running through the gamut of lunge and step-up variations, and you'll never think to ask questions like those.

Alwyn includes the step-up in the single-leg-stance category, separate from the other lower-body movements. It's not an immediately intuitive choice. The squat, hinge, and lunge are distinct movement patterns, whereas the single-leg exercises are derived from those movement patterns but involve balancing on one leg while performing them.

The category includes step-ups, as noted, along with single-leg squat and deadlift variations. At one level, these exercises are just good muscle builders, forcing you to move most of your body weight, along with some kind of external resistance, using one leg at a time.

But if that's all they did, they wouldn't be worth their own category. You'll always be able to move more weight with both feet on the floor and your body stabilized. Single-leg exercises add a unique stability-mobility challenge. You must stabilize your ankle when you're standing on one leg. You also have to stabilize your core with full mobility in your hip joints. If you have any weakness anywhere in the movement chain, from floor to core, it'll be exposed in a single-leg exercise.

The one thing they're bad for is your ego. If you've spent any time watching training videos on YouTube, particularly from kettlebell specialists, you'll feel really bad about yourself when you try to match the range of motion they achieve on single-leg squats. Worse, you'll probably get hurt if you push too far, too fast. Single-leg exercises work best if you progress carefully, gradually increasing your range of motion and the amount of weight you use. Few of us have the combination of strength, mobility, and stability to impress people with our form on the most advanced exercises. It takes a long time to get there; by that point, you'll have impressed yourself, which is what matters most.

Now, having mentioned mobility and stability, let's move on to discuss those and the other fitness qualities that improve your physique, your performance, and perhaps most important of all, your lifelong health.

# All Fitness Is Muscular Fitness

I GOT MY FIRST PERSONAL-TRAINING CERTIFICATION in 1997 from the American Council on Exercise. On page 2 of the textbook, we were told that optimum fitness has these three components:

- Cardiovascular endurance
- Muscular strength and flexibility
- Ideal body weight

It seemed to make sense at the time. Today it just looks . . . random. I mean, who puts strength and flexibility on the same line? Cardiovascular health and fitness are obviously important, but what does "cardiovascular endurance" mean? Are we talking about a threshold level of aerobic fitness, enough to complete a workout, play your favorite sport, or survive a twenty-mile hike with your local Boy Scout troop? Training for an endurance sport? Or do we mean that vague category of moving-for-the-sake-of-moving exercise we call "cardio"? Finally, is "ideal body weight" a worthwhile goal? Wouldn't it make more sense to focus on body *composition*, with a goal of increasing your muscle mass while lowering your body-fat percentage?

These aren't idle questions. As our friend Dan John says, if something is important, you should work on it every time you train. The NROL standard for a training session is sixty minutes, max. So whatever Alwyn decides is important enough to train, that's what you're going to work on within that one-hour window, three times a week.

The traditionalist view of fitness is that you need to do some of everything, regardless of what you hope to accomplish with your workouts. A man most interested in increasing muscle size and strength would be told he also needs to do steady-pace endurance exercise several days a week, even though it wouldn't help him reach his goals, and might actually work against them. A woman focused mainly on weight loss would be encouraged to invest time in stretching, which back then was pushed as an elaborate, time-consuming, muscle-by-muscle process. How would ten to fifteen minutes of stretching help someone shed fat, especially if that time could be used for exercises that improve mobility while also burning a lot of calories and perhaps building muscle as well?

Alwyn ditched that some-of-everything paradigm a long time ago. Like many trainers I met in the late nineties and early 2000s, he didn't think he was giving his clients fair value if he put them on a treadmill to run while he stood there watching. If he was getting paid to train someone, he was going to *train* her. That is, he was going to teach her how to do the exercises, coach her through a routine that offered increasing challenges, and keep her moving for the entire session. (I use the female pronoun on purpose. Alwyn has always trained his female clients to build strength and muscle as a path to making them leaner and lighter.)

He also encouraged and expected his clients to do other types of exercise on their own. That worked fine until the mid to late 2000s, when he and his trainers at Results Fitness noticed that their clients were no longer doing much outside the gym. If they were exercising, it tended to be repetitive, unbalanced activities, in some cases creating or exacerbating issues with strength, mobility, or core stability.

Today Alwyn and his trainers look to develop six key aspects of muscular fitness in every training session:

- Joint mobility, aka range of motion
- Core stability

- Balance and coordination
- Power
- Strength
- Metabolic conditioning

Each of those is important. But how important would any be, to the exclusion of the others? And more important, does it matter if you separate them at all? Indulge me as I rule on that.

**NEW RULE #11** ○ **The lines between "strength," "cardio," and "flexibility" aren't as clear as you think.**

When I showed Alwyn the circa-1997 ACE definition of fitness, the first thing he pointed out was the assumption that there are clear delineations, suggesting that for one to begin another must end. So jogging is one thing, heavy lifting is another, and flexibility is something else entirely.

But what happens when you do a grueling set of step-ups that includes fifteen repetitions with each leg? You're certainly developing strength; you should be able to use slightly heavier weights almost every time you repeat the workout. You're also developing muscular endurance. If you stuck with the same weight, you'd soon be able to do many more repetitions than you could at first. The harder you push yourself to increase your performance—the combined improvements in strength and endurance—the harder you'll work your cardiorespiratory system, which has to pump blood to the working muscles. In fact, you'll challenge all three of your body's energy systems by the time you finish the set. (See Sidebar on page 25.)

Now think of what happens when you begin Alwyn's warm-up routine. Some of you will be huffing and puffing, if you aren't used to those exercises and techniques, a pretty good sign that you're training something. But what? It's not traditional cardio exercise, because you're only doing a few repetitions of each exercise before moving on to the next. It's not traditional stretching, since you're rarely stopping to hold your body in a fixed position so you can stretch specific muscles to their full length. Instead, you're moving lots of muscles in and out of those stretched positions, with an emphasis on *moving*. Many of these exercises challenge your balance, which means you're developing strength in muscles that aren't used to the new movements.

Can you find the point where strength training begins, or cardio exercise ends, or flexibility takes precedence over the other two?

## Who Has the Energy for This?

"Energy" is one of our favorite words in the fitness industry. Magazines and websites love to use it in headlines like "Get more energy!" (Always with an exclamation point! Why? Because it's more energetic that way!) Gyms across the country are named Energy Fitness. There's even a stimulant product advertised on TV called 5-hour Energy.

Ask a nutritionist what energy is, and she won't need many words, or much punctuation. It's food. Period. When she talks about energy going in or going out of your body, she means the calories you eat vs. the calories you burn off. Thus, a nutritionist would see irony in a health club—a place to *burn* calories—promising that its patrons will somehow *receive* energy by training there. Energy Steakhouse—*that's* where you'd go to load up. Energy Drain would be an accurate name for a gym, although the investors would probably rule it out.

The human body has three ways to turn food into movement, called *energy systems*. The first is your aerobic energy system. You of course know that "aerobic" means "with oxygen." You use oxygen every minute of every day to tap into your abundant supplies of fat and carbohydrate. (A healthy body at rest will burn more than 50 percent fat.) During exercise, the ratio gradually shifts; the harder you work, the higher the percentage of carbohydrate you use for fuel.

You also have two anaerobic energy systems, which you use during more intense exercise. For a near-maximum lift or all-out sprint, your body calls on the phosphagen system, which uses adenosine triphosphate (ATP) and creatine phosphate (CP). Your body has enough ready-made ATP and CP for about ten seconds' worth of extreme exertion. Once you've hit your limit, the phosphagen system shuts down while your body replenishes its ATP and CP.

The other anaerobic system is called glycolysis. Since you only have a small amount of ATP and quickly run out of it, this system creates more by splitting apart molecules of glycogen, which is the storage form of carbohydrate. The process lowers the pH of your blood, leaving your muscles feeling fatigued. Few of us can use this system for more than a minute or two at a time.

Your body typically uses these three systems concurrently whenever you're up and moving.

## NEW RULE #12 • The benefits of the program exceed the sum of the individual parts.

Let's return to the American Council on Exercise definition of fitness. Back then I still believed you weren't truly "fit" unless you ordered everything on the menu. I didn't enjoy endurance exercise, and I can produce credible witnesses to the fact I wasn't good at it. But I did it because I thought I was supposed to.

Today I think there's a stronger case to be made for doing the type of exercise you enjoy most, doing it consistently and with as much vigor and ambition as you can muster, and letting your health take care of itself. If all you like to do is walk, get out and walk hard, as the great Dewey Cox sang. While you're at it, walk long. Walk fast too, or at least vary your speed from time to time. Walk up and down hills, and get off the path to walk across uneven terrain.

Same goes for yoga, or golf, or anything else. If it's all you're willing to try, at least try a lot of it. Sitting is the most dangerous thing we do, and most of us do it for hours a day. Anything that gets you up out of your chair and onto your feet is better than nothing. Not-nothing is the number-one benefit of any fitness program. Not-nothing burns (some) calories, increases your metabolism (slightly and transiently), develops endurance in the muscles you use (but only those muscles), and probably improves other fitness qualities like balance, coordination, and the speed at which you can do specific movements.

If not-nothing leads you to a true, consistent exercise routine, you're guaranteed to improve your cardiovascular fitness, your insulin sensitivity (that is, your ability to clear sugar out of your bloodstream efficiently), your immune system, your mood, and the strength and function of whatever parts of your musculoskeletal system you use in the activity. If you run, for example, you're going to develop greater lower-body bone density. You'll almost certainly live longer, and in better overall health as well.

Alwyn's *Supercharged* workouts cross the not-nothing barrier the minute you enter your workout space and begin the warm-up exercises. Fifty to sixty minutes later, you're in the "pretty much everything" zone. You've burned a lot of calories, cranked up your metabolic rate so high that it'll take hours to return to normal, moved all your joints through their full range of motion, and forced all your major muscles to work both hard and long, building strength and endurance. Since you've done all this with careful attention to your posture and form, you've improved your core stability. And because you've included exercises that challenge your balance and coordination, you've improved those qualities as well. You'll breathe hard as you push your muscles to exhaustion on the strength exercises. (If you aren't, you're doing them wrong.)

All that is a prelude to the workout's final component: metabolic training. You'll choose from a long list of drills shown in Chapter 16, any of which push you to finish the workout with lots of movement in lots of directions, challenging your endurance and fortitude in ever-shifting ratios.

The workout covers every aspect of muscular fitness. Since the heart is a muscle, responsible for pumping blood to all those other muscles, it gets trained along with everything else. You don't have to worry about mundane, steady-pace cardio exercise, unless it's something you enjoy (in which case I apologize for calling it "mundane"). You won't have to worry about long, boring stretching routines, unless you like to do them. (You still have to admit they're pretty boring.) A few months of these workouts and you'll be in better shape, however you define it: leaner, more muscular, stronger, better conditioned, more athletic and coordinated. Work hard enough for long enough, and you can be "fit" by any reasonable definition.

What I can't say is what any single part of the workout can do without all the other parts.

Take strength, for example. In previous books I've mentioned studies showing that physical strength correlates with longevity. But the elderly men and women in those studies—typically recruited in retirement communities—aren't lifters. The stronger ones aren't exactly "strong"; they just haven't lost as much strength as their peers.

Or take the idea that strength training improves athletic performance. I don't think you'll find a coach who claims it doesn't, but proof is harder to pin down than you'd expect. Strength can be correlated to improved speed and all sorts of linear things, like throwing harder or kicking farther. But does it help improve the skills that win games? Does it help you put the ball into the net (assuming you're not playing tennis, where that wouldn't be good at all)?

The research, it turns out, isn't conclusive. The entire strength and conditioning field may believe the stronger athlete is the better athlete, and I'm certainly inclined to agree with them. But studies have turned up limited evidence that even a large increase in strength and power translates to a measurable improvement in on-field performance.

Another example: Wake me up in the middle of the night, far from the nearest research database, and ask me if balance is key to athletic performance. I'm going to say yes, right after I yell at you for ripping me out of a sound sleep to ask such a silly question. But is it silly?

When Con Hrysomallis, a researcher at Victoria University in Australia, looked at a vast body of research, he noted a link to injury risk (better balance = fewer injuries), but "the relationship between balance ability and athletic performance is less clear." To no one's surprise, gymnasts have the best balance among athletes. However, in surfing and judo—both of which would seem to require otherworldly balance—there was no link to performance. The best didn't have better balance than their less skilled peers. He concluded that balance training could help regular people like us more than it helps elite athletes.

You may not realize you're training your balance in Alwyn's workouts, beyond the times when you're doing single-leg exercises and you're acutely aware of the risk of toppling over. But from beginning to end, you're pushed out of your comfort cocoon, forced to move in new directions, hold yourself steady in unique positions, and from time to time move unbalanced loads.

We know all that is "good," and way better than *not* challenging your body to learn new movements and skills. We just can't say how much it helps outside the context of the full program.

But there may be one aspect of muscular fitness that surpasses the others in life-long importance.

## NEW RULE #13  •  Power is to fitness as fitness is to health.

The difference between strength and power is easy to distinguish on a metaphorical level. Strength is demonstrable, but power works best when you can't see how people use it to get what they want. In physiology, it's a lot more explicit. Strength is the ability to exert force. Power is force multiplied by velocity. Put more simply, strength is what you can lift, and power is the speed at which you can lift it.

There's a sliding scale for power. The smaller the object, the faster you can move it, but the less power your body generates to make it move. Power peaks when you lift something that's about 70 percent of your maximum. So if you're a woman who can squat 100 pounds once with good form, you would express peak muscle power when you squat 70 pounds as fast as you can. If you're a guy who can deadlift 300 pounds, your power would peak, more or less, when you pull 200 pounds off the floor at max velocity.

The four Basic Training programs in *Supercharged* have a specific power-training component. Most of us have little opportunity to move fast in our daily routines, and health-club chains have done all of us a disservice by convincing their members to work out on machines, which force you to go at a slower pace and punish you for going faster. Doing something fast every workout reminds us of how much fun it is to run and jump and throw things around.

But the more advanced programs don't include that specific training category. Studies are pretty clear that when athletes train for maximum power (moving lighter weights at top speed) or maximum strength (moving heavier weights at any speed) they get about the same improvements in jumping and sprinting. The researchers concluded that, over time, the overall benefits of strength training would exceed those of power training. So if you can increase power by training for strength, but you can't increase strength to the same degree by training for power, it makes more sense to focus on strength.

For the youngest readers, these distinctions between strength and power aren't all that crucial. It's still important to do the exercises as part of Basic Training, since they contribute to the overall conditioning you'll need for the Hypertrophy and Strength & Power programs. But you aren't yet at any particular risk of losing the power you already have. It's a different story for those of us old enough to remember when the continents were a single land mass.

We know that adults lose muscle as we age, and when we lose muscle we would expect to see drops in strength, power, and any number of performance variables, like walking speed. But when researchers at Tufts University looked at adults in their seventies, they found that power loss occurred at several times the rate of strength loss. And strength loss was itself three times faster than muscle loss, which was about 2 percent per year.

It's not the loss of muscle in general that puts you into that wheelchair. It's the loss of Type II muscle fibers, which generate four times the power of endurance-oriented Type I fibers. Those fibers come in bundles, called motor units, and each motor unit has a nerve cell to switch it on when needed. When you lose motor units, you also lose nerve cells. Lose nerve cells and you lose abilities.

One of the Tufts studies compared a group of healthy, middle-aged adults to two groups of men and women in their seventies—one healthy, one with mobility limitations. The latter group had 25 percent less muscle than the middle-aged people, but 95 percent less lower-body power. Compared to their nonlimited peers—also in their seventies—they had 13 percent less muscle, but 65 percent less power.

That's where the death spiral begins: The loss of Type II motor units precipitates a higher magnitude of strength loss, and an even more dramatic power drain. No matter what age you happen to be as you read this, remember that the goal is to get old without getting feeble. That's just as true at the start of adult life as it is in retirement. All of us, young and old, need to pay attention to our body's most precious resource: our Type II muscle fibers.

As luck would have it, that's the subject of the next chapter.

# PART 2

# YOUR MUSCLES, YOURSELF

# Bigger Is Better

IN A 2010 PAPER in the *Journal of Strength and Conditioning Research*, author and trainer Brad Schoenfeld showed that lifting makes muscles bigger in three primary ways:

- Mechanical tension—that is, stress imposed on muscles and connective tissues
- Muscle damage—the small tears and distortions you create through the combination of mechanical tension and swelling from fluids entering the muscle
- Metabolic stress—the result of anaerobic glycolysis (described in Chapter 3), which leaves your body swimming with lactic acid and other by-products of difficult exercise

The volume of training also plays a role, Schoenfeld explained in a follow-up article in *Strength and Conditioning Journal*, although it's a bit of a wild card. More seems to be better, but we can't say if it's because your muscles are under more tension, are under tension longer, sustain more damage, induce more metabolic stress, or swell with pride because you give them so much love.

Another wild card: All these factors are highly variable from one individual to the next. We'll start the ruling there, and then explore what we know and don't know about making our favorite biological system even more magnificent to behold.

## NEW RULE #14 • The muscle fairy has a sick sense of humor.

Researchers at the University of Alabama at Birmingham found a way to predict which of us will add the most muscle when we begin a workout program. Those who have the most satellite cells—these are stem cells attached to the membranes of muscle fibers; when needed, they can help muscle cells grow or repair themselves—will be "extreme responders" to a training program, even if they've never lifted before. (None of the subjects in the study had trained for at least five years.) They achieved growth of more than 50 percent in the targeted muscles. Those labeled "nonresponders" started out with the fewest satellite cells per muscle fiber, and they achieved zero growth. None. Twelve weeks of strength training, and all they got was a stupid T-shirt.

In between were "moderate responders," who made up about half of the study population. The other half was divided evenly between extreme responders and those who were S.O.L.

This probably matches your own experience. Whether you're young or old, male or female, if you're a longtime lifter you've known a few people whose first whiff of sweat and chalk dust caused their biceps to swell up like pregnant rodents. We now know it's because the deck was stacked in their favor from birth. It's the physiological equivalent of a trust fund, with one string attached: They have to lift to see the benefits.

Alas, for every winner in the genetic lottery, there's someone who has to work twice as hard to get any measureable results.

Yes, it sucks, and no, it's not fair.

## NEW RULE #15 • Every program is a hypertrophy program.

Want to make your muscles grow? Find something you need both hands to lift. Lift it, and keep lifting it until your muscles can't do another repetition. Set it down. Rest. Repeat twice.

Stupid? Sure. But if you do this stupid workout three times a week for, say, ten weeks, the muscles you use *will* get bigger.

That was the conclusion of Stuart Phillips and his research team at McMaster

University in Ontario. They had untrained lifters work out for ten weeks using either a light weight (30 percent of their one-repetition maximum) for three sets or a heavy weight (80 percent of their 1RM) for either one or three sets. To make sure the results weren't skewed by high or low responders, they used just one exercise—the leg extension—and had their subjects use a different system for each leg. Thus, if you took part in this study, you might do three sets with a light weight with your left leg, and one set with a heavy weight with your right leg.

To the surprise of almost everyone who studies these things, the weight didn't make any difference. Volume mattered—the legs that did three sets gained more than twice as much muscle size as the legs that did a single set—but heavy and light weights offered about the same benefits, more or less. (Those using heavy weights saw more growth in Type II fibers, while Type I fibers grew more with lighter weights. But overall hypertrophy was statistically similar.)

The protocol is even crazier than the pick-up-anything-and-lift-it program I described a minute ago. But the researchers aren't crazy; they're just willing to do experiments no one else would attempt for results few of us are willing to believe.

The lesson here is simple enough: You can build muscle with light weights, heavy weights, and everything in between, as long as you create mechanical tension, muscle damage, and metabolic stress. But the *application* of the lesson would be a monumental pain in the ass. There's only one way to create enough tension, damage, and metabolic stress to build muscle with a puny weight: Lift until your muscles can't lift it anymore. The subjects in the study did 30 to 40 repetitions per set. Even worse, they did three sets per workout and three workouts per week for ten weeks. That's just one exercise with one leg. Can you imagine how tedious it would be if your entire program worked like that? (Since the researchers used novices in the study, we don't know if trained lifters would get the same results, even if they were tempted to try it.)

Alwyn's programs include some high-rep training—as many as 20 per set for several workouts in Hypertrophy I, and 15 per set at different points. I used to dread those workouts, racing through the sets to get it over with. I still don't like them, but knowing they have a purpose gives me incentive to take them seriously.

Which brings me to . . .

## NEW RULE #16 • Every program is a strength program.

Let's talk numbers for a moment. Imagine an exercise in which your one-rep max is 100 pounds. For some of you that might be a deadlift; for others it might be a one-arm, no-look, behind-the-back biceps curl. It doesn't really matter for the point I want to make. Here's a quick guide to the weights you would most likely use for the rep ranges Alwyn prescribes in *Supercharged*:

| Reps per set | Estimated weight/percentage of 1-rep max |
|:---:|:---:|
| 2 | 95 |
| 3 | 93 |
| 4 | 90 |
| 5 | 87 |
| 6 | 85 |
| 8 | 80 |
| 10 | 75 |
| 12 | 67 |
| 15 | 65 |
| 20 | 55* |

Source: *Essentials of Strength Training and Conditioning*, second edition.
*Just a guess; the chart stops at 15 reps.

Studies have shown that lifters typically choose weights that are too light to get the results they want. Perfect example: In a study published in 2008, researchers at the College of New Jersey recruited young women with, on average, about four years' worth of lifting experience. The women were told to do sets of 10 reps of some common exercises. The chart above shows that a lifter who wanted to reach exhaustion by the final rep would need to use about 75 percent of her one-rep max.

The subjects were divided into two groups. The ones who worked with personal trainers selected weights that were *barely half* of their one-rep max. In other words, they chose weights for sets of 10 that would've been appropriate for sets of 20. But the ones who didn't work with trainers did even worse. They chose weights that were, on average, 42.3 percent of their max on those exercises.

A similar study at Grand Valley State University in Michigan used a mixed group of young men and women. These were beginners, half of whom were given detailed instructions on selecting appropriate weights; the other half were simply shown how to use the exercise machines. The group with instruction used slightly heavier weights, but both groups stopped well short of exhaustion on all exercises. Most participants ended their sets at or near 12 reps, even when their weights were just 50 to 60 percent of their max.

Two points:

- Almost every set of every workout, whether you're using high reps, low reps, or anything in between, should be *somewhat* exhausting. Sometimes you have to use the first set, or even the first two sets, to figure out the right weight for that rep range. But the final set should always take your muscles pretty close to their limit.
- The second time you do that workout—that is, the same exercises for the same sets and reps—you should work with heavier weights on most of the exercises, if not all of them. Or you can shoot for more reps with the same weight, if you fell short in the first workout. So if you completed 10 reps when the workout called for 12, or 12 when your goal was 15, you want to get more reps before you increase the weight.

Put another way, you want proof that you're getting stronger from one workout to the next. This is your one benchmark, the only sure way to know that your program is working, and that you're making it work.

## NEW RULE #17 • Every program is a fat-loss program.

A good strength workout triggers a chain reaction that's almost biblical in its complexity: this begets that, that begets something else, and something else begets yet another hormone or enzyme that permits more protein to enter muscle cells, or less protein to break down and leave, or both.

Over time, this reaction to the cellular and metabolic stress imposed by training leaves you with bigger, stronger, better-fueled muscles. But in the short term—the hours and days immediately following each workout—your metabolism speeds up. It has to. You're asking it to do things it doesn't ordinarily do. That means it has to use fuel it doesn't ordinarily use. *When your goal is fat loss, that's exactly what you want.*

It's also what you want when you're trying to build muscle. Which brings us to perhaps the most important concept in this book: The goal of training is to force your body to make adaptations. Good programs, like Alwyn's, give you the framework. But it's still up to you to make the adaptations occur. You have to push yourself to use heavier weights from one workout to the next, which increases mechanical tension on your muscles. That makes them bigger as well as stronger. You also push yourself to get a bit more done from workout to workout, which increases metabolic stress. That not only creates a cascade of hormonal and chemical reactions to make your muscles bigger, it increases your metabolic rate as your body repairs the damage, and improves your overall conditioning as well.

That's why good workouts are hard workouts. They don't accomplish much if they aren't.

## WHAT WE KNOW, AND DON'T KNOW, ABOUT MUSCLE GROWTH

There's an unwritten rule—an oral tradition, I guess—that says anyone who writes about strength training must, at some point in his career, mention Milo of Croton. He was a real guy, a famed wrestler in Greece in the sixth century B.C., and an Olympic champion in the original context. Milo's daily diet is said to have included twenty pounds of meat, twenty pounds of bread, and eighteen pints of wine. The meat and bread alone would've been about 34,000 calories, or almost triple the 12,000 daily calories swimmer Michael Phelps was rumored to eat while training for the Olympics in 2008. (Phelps later denied the story, saying "it's pretty much impossible" for anyone to eat that much.)

But the reason Milo is brought up so often today, more than 2,500 years later, is a load of bull. Legend says that he started carrying the bull around as a calf, and his strength increased along with the bull's weight. By the time it was fully grown, he could still lift it.

Consider the improbability: A calf today typically weighs about 80 pounds, and gains about 2.5 pounds per day. An adult bull weighs between 2,000 and 3,000 pounds, with testicles measuring 16 inches in circumference. The biggest, strongest powerlifters today, with the benefits of steroids and specialized lifting gear, can squat a little over a thousand pounds. Strongman competitors have an event called the yoke walk—it's exactly what it sounds like: walking while supporting a super-heavy weight across your shoulders—in which, again, a thousand pounds is a pretty big deal. What are the odds that anyone in ancient Greece was two or three times as strong as one of them?

In fairness, Milo's feat isn't brought up for its veracity. It's used as an example of the power of progressive resistance. No matter how weak you are when you begin, you'll be much stronger after years of dedicated training, thanks to small, incremental increases in the loads you lift.

Let's start there.

## Mechanical tension

The Milo story gets one thing right: You increase tension over time by using progressively heavier weights. But it gets just about everything else wrong, starting with the strategy.

Strength tends to increase rapidly at the start of a program, thanks to your muscles and nerves learning to coordinate themselves in new ways. There's little actual hypertrophy. But once muscle growth begins, the biggest gains, again, come right away. Studies have shown increases of 10 to 15 percent in the first three to four months of training. They slow down considerably after that. There's a tiny window in which Milo's strength curve would match the bull's growth curve, but it wouldn't last long.

Moreover, walking around with a relatively light load, like an eighty-pound calf, wouldn't stimulate your Type II muscle fibers, which are responsible for strength and power performance, and would offer more benefit to an athlete like Milo.

Remember that all of them are arranged in motor units—a bundle of fibers and the nerve cell that tells them when to switch on or off. The size principle, a basic law of exercise science, says that motor units are recruited from smallest to largest. So when you lift a near-maximum load, you activate all your motor units. The other way to activate a significant number of Type II motor units is to work with lighter weights to the point of muscular exhaustion. The Type II units are forced to participate when Type I units become fatigued.

You may wonder why any intermediate or advanced lifter would bother using lighter weights. If all the motor units work when you lift heavy weights with low reps, why not do that almost all the time, on almost every exercise? That's a good strategy if your goal is maximum strength. But for hypertrophy, it's not, as we'll see in the next section.

## Time under tension

Imagine yourself doing an all-out set of your favorite exercise—let's say 5 reps—with a really heavy weight. Of course you aren't going to do those reps at a deliberately moderate speed. You're going to knock them out. The entire set might last five to ten seconds. Now lower the weight and do the same exercise, but this time slow down your tempo so a set of 10 reps lasts 30 seconds. Your muscles are shaking and swollen by the end of the set, your breath is labored, and your heart is pounding. A day or two later, the muscles are stiff and sore. If they happen to be lower-body muscles, you feel like a robot every time you get up to walk to the restroom.

What happened?

- You hit your muscles with a unique training stimulus, which induced more muscle damage than usual.
- Because you slowed down your repetitions, you forced your muscles to spend more time lengthening. We call that the negative or eccentric part of the lift. It's associated with more muscle damage, and also with greater muscle growth.
- The extended time under tension would also increase the amount of energy used through anaerobic glycolysis, which is not only linked to increased metabolic stress, but also to more energy used both during and after the training session.

Nobody can say just how much time under tension is ideal. Focus on it too much and you end up doing all your training with lighter weights at slower speeds, which is not only boring, it limits your development of absolute strength and power. Those still matter, because the stronger you are, the more you should be able to lift with any system of sets and reps.

## Less Blood, More Muscle?

If you've heard of hypoxia, which occurs when some or all of your body is deprived of oxygen, it's probably in the context of a serious condition like altitude sickness. A small but fascinating body of research shows that it can also be a potent muscle-building tool. Japanese researchers, who call it Kaatsu training, tested it on elderly subjects by having them do biceps curls with light weights and their blood flow cut off, and compared them to subjects who worked the same muscles with moderate weights and full blood flow. The occluded subjects and the ones using moderate weights saw similar increases in muscle size. Both those groups gained more than the group using light weights without restriction.

You don't need to cut off your own blood flow to benefit from the hypoxic effect. With more time under tension, swelling within the targeted muscles will limit blood flow, giving you the one-two punch of muscle damage and metabolic stress. That will be followed by increased blood flow afterward, which will put more nutrients into the muscles. The combination should also lead to a higher post-workout metabolic rate.

Alwyn likes to focus on time under tension in two contexts: acute and chronic. The former is how much time it takes to finish each individual set. The second is the cumulative time under tension in a workout, or even a series of workouts. You'll see this applied in the Strength & Power programs. You'll do several sets with heavy weights and low reps, and then finish with longer sets using lighter weights. That way you employ all the mechanisms linked to muscle hypertrophy without sacrificing top-end strength and power.

## Variety

One more whack at poor old Milo: Doing the same exercise over and over for years is not an ideal way to increase muscle size. If you're a strength athlete—a powerlifter or Strongman competitor—of course you have to practice the lifts. Your goal is to groove the movement pattern and make it as efficient as possible. But if you're more interested in appearance than performance, the last thing you want is to focus so much on the same lifts that you miss out on the muscle damage and metabolic stress that would come from changing things up and doing unfamiliar movements.

Two more reasons to change up exercises regularly:

- Different angles employ different muscles in different ways. As Brad Schoenfeld wrote in the *Journal of Strength and Conditioning Research*, "Given the need to fully stimulate all fibers within a muscle, it would seem that a frequent exercise rotation is warranted to maximize the hypertrophic response."
- Any powerlifter will tell you that the downside to grooving a movement is an injury mechanism called *pattern overload*. Changing the direction of force, however slightly, gives your joints some relief.

Everything mentioned in this chapter is influenced by your diet, particularly the amount, type, and timing of protein. Turn the page, and we'll dive in.

# The Care and Feeding of Your Muscles

How to be a musclehead in four easy steps:

1. Lift weights.
2. Eat lots of protein.
3. Tell everyone you know about how you lift weights and eat lots of protein.
4. Start a blog about lifting weights and eating lots of protein.

The "lifting weights" part is nonnegotiable. Alwyn has helped shift the methods somewhat, from the old bodybuilding model of long workouts focused on individual muscles to the NROL emphasis on total-body strength and performance. But just about all of us agree that muscle development depends on the three factors I described in Chapter 4: mechanical tension, muscle damage, and metabolic stress, with the most emphasis on the first one. If you push yourself to use heavier weights over time, and you work your muscles to or near exhaustion on most of your sets, Alwyn's system takes care of the rest. You'll get plenty of metabolic stress (it's his fiendish specialty), and muscle damage will occur with hard work and a variety of exercises.

But protein . . . well, that's more nuanced than we once thought.

## NEW RULE #18 • Muscle building takes place every hour of every day.

For most of my lifting life I've focused on post-workout nutrition: getting a whole lot of protein into my stomach as soon as possible. If I gave pre-workout nutrition any thought, it was mostly to make sure I had something in my stomach so the hunger pangs wouldn't distract me.

Recent research suggests that the total amount of protein you get throughout the day is far more important than what you have immediately before or after a single workout. This is something my friend Alan Aragon, a nutritionist, has been saying for several years: If you give your body the raw materials it needs, with sufficient volume and quality, timing becomes much less important.

I don't want to say that timing takes care of itself; it's still a good idea to eat a protein-rich meal an hour or two before training, and to go out of your way to consume high-quality protein within an hour after you finish, or two hours at the most. The protein in your muscles breaks down rapidly during and after strength training. Starve them and the net effect is a wasted workout. But with a daily diet that gives your muscles plenty to work with, timing becomes less urgent.

The one exception is if you train first thing in the morning, before eating breakfast. Your body will already be in a catabolic state—breaking down muscle protein—and your workout will only accelerate that process. A post-workout shake with at least 20 grams of whey protein will put your body in an anabolic state—building new muscle tissue—and a protein-rich meal within an hour or two of training will seal the deal . . . as long as you eat normally the rest of the day.

## NEW RULE #19 • A new lifter needs more protein than a weight-room veteran.

The longtime lifter, male or female, understands the importance of protein to recover from one workout to the next, and we understand that recovery is the key to making new gains. Those are hard enough to achieve after years under the bar, and most of us would rather err on the side of excess rather than risk depriving our bodies of raw materials.

The inexperienced lifter, conversely, will typically take a wait-and-see approach. First he'll want to know if his body responds to the workouts. When it does, he assumes that whatever he's been eating is good enough. It usually takes years of lifting, with those newbie gains deep in the rearview mirror, to realize his diet isn't optimal for a lifter. So he increases his protein in a dramatic way, including a post-workout shake, while cutting back on fat and/or carbs. Almost overnight his muscles start growing again. His waist probably shrinks as well.

He tells himself that he's learned a valuable lesson: a sloppy, low-protein diet is fine for a beginner, but it takes a lot more protein once you're a true musclehead. Soon he starts a blog and creates a Facebook fan page to share this revealed truth with his fellow lifters.

Unfortunately, it's the wrong lesson.

Some research has shown that experienced lifters use protein more efficiently than novices, with a smaller anabolic window following a workout—twenty-four hours, vs. forty-eight hours for the beginner. Muscles respond to protein faster in the advanced lifter, and it takes less protein to get a maximum response.

I like this analogy from Stuart Phillips of McMaster University, whose lab has performed many of the studies mentioned in this section of *Supercharged*: "Think of your muscles as a bag. When we're novices the bag is not as full, and there's more room to store protein. When you're more experienced your bag's a little fuller. Adaptations/changes/gains don't come so easily." You still have to eat high-quality protein, he adds, and time some of it around your workouts, but quantity matters a bit less than it does for the novice.

The message here is simple enough: Every lifter—newbies and gym rats, male and female, young and old—benefits from the combination of strength training and dietary protein. Trying to build muscle without a protein-rich diet is like Robin fighting crime without Batman. He's going to get his butt stomped, with no measurable benefit to the citizens of Gotham.

## NEW RULE #20 ◦ The older you are, the more protein you need.

If a newbie lifter in his twenties is unlikely to seek out extra protein when it would help most, imagine the dilemma of the AARP-eligible novice. Not only is he out of his comfort zone in the gym, for much of his life he's heard "experts" in the media telling us our bones will shrivel and our kidneys will implode if we seek out any protein beyond our current intake. He's already biased against the concept.

But older lifters have two big mechanisms working against them: First, their muscles have developed anabolic resistance. That is, their bodies are reluctant to use dietary protein to build new muscle tissue. Second, the hormone insulin doesn't work as well as it does in younger lifters to prevent muscle tissue from breaking down during and after a workout. New research from Phillips's team at McMaster shows that it takes twice as much post-workout protein to reach the point of saturation, when their muscles have as much as they can use. That's 40 grams of whey protein for older lifters, vs. 20 grams for younger ones.

The studies used male lifters, so it's unclear if these numbers work for women (more on gender in the next section). Also unclear is the point at which anabolic resistance begins. The studies compared men in their twenties to men in their seventies. What about those of us in our fifties? Should we split the difference and use 30 grams of post-workout protein as our guideline? Alas, we just don't know yet.

But there's plenty we do know.

## DO MEN AND WOMEN USE PROTEIN THE SAME WAY?

According to a new textbook called *Dietary Protein and Resistance Exercise*, rates of protein synthesis are about the same for young men and women, when the researchers adjust for the differences in total lean mass—that is, muscle, bone, and everything else that isn't fat. Results are similar when comparing young and middle-aged lifters of both genders—although, as noted, nobody can really say where you draw the line between "middle" and "old" age, or when your muscles need more protein to get the same response.

Studies haven't detected differences in protein synthesis for women based on their menstrual cycle, although women with menstrual disorders may not get the same results from training as their more regular counterparts, due to a blunted hormonal response to training.

## HOW MUCH DO YOU NEED?

The government-approved minimum protein requirement for adults is crazy low: 0.8 gram per kilogram (2.2 pounds) of body weight per day. That's about 66 grams per day for a 180-pounder like me. For a 130-pound woman, it's 47 grams, and for that 220-pounder who just got kicked out of Planet Fitness for having visible neck veins, it's just 80 grams—basically, a couple of chicken breasts. This I can guarantee: If you do Alwyn's workouts while eating a similarly minuscule amount of protein, you're going to lose muscle and look and feel much worse.

What's a better target? The simplest path is to double the minimum. I don't know if I would *thrive* on 132 grams a day, but I doubt if I would lose muscle. If you're cutting the overall calories in your diet while doing Alwyn's programs, I recommend the old bodybuilding standby: 1 gram of protein per pound of body weight per day.

Aragon has a more elegant twist on that recommendation: 1 gram per pound of *target* body weight. So if you weigh 145 and you're trying to lose ten, shoot for 135 grams a day.

## WHEN DO YOU NEED IT?

Immediately after a workout, as I mentioned, the protein in your muscles is breaking down at an accelerated pace. "Breakdown" sounds bad, but as a recent paper in *Nutrition and Metabolism* explains, it probably leaves us with better overall muscle quality by getting rid of damaged bits, which will be replaced (and then some) by newer, healthier proteins. That process, called protein synthesis, is happening 100 to 150 percent faster than normal.

Given those two phenomena—accelerated breakdown and accumulation—you'd think that it's crucial to get post-workout protein into your stomach ASAP. That's what early studies showed, and it's what muscleheads like us believed for a generation. What we didn't consider is that many of those studies used subjects who were training on an empty stomach. Not only that, they compared lifters who got protein to control subjects who got either a noncaloric placebo or straight carbohydrates. Another issue: some studies used untrained lifters, some didn't.

We now know (with apologies for repeating myself) that well-fed, experienced lifters don't get the same boost from a post-workout protein shake. Total daily protein intake matters most, as long as you're getting some of it within an hour or two on both sides of your workouts.

For beginners? I lean toward the old-school recommendation of a protein shake immediately after training. If nothing else, it reminds you to feed your muscles. It's like watering your garden in the spring. You know the plants won't grow without water, and you're never sure if nature is providing enough rain. So you break out the sprinkler, just in case. Moreover, it ensures that you get at least one powerful dose of the best muscle-building nutrients we have (more on that in a bit).

Research shows that 20 to 25 grams of post-workout protein maximizes protein synthesis, with the previously noted exception of elderly lifters, who max out with around 40 grams. There's no danger to consuming more, but there's also no benefit. Your body will simply excrete the excess, although it might use some of it for energy.

Nutritionist Mike Roussell uses a light-switch analogy. Once you flip on a light switch, you can't turn it on more to make the room brighter. It's the same with protein synthesis. Once you've flipped the switch—the combination of strength training and post-workout protein—you've done all you can. More protein beyond the amount known to maximize the effect won't help.

## WHAT TYPES ARE BEST FOR LIFTERS?

All protein sources include a mix of amino acids, the building blocks of protein. There are twenty amino acids, of which nine are considered "essential," meaning your body can't make them out of other aminos. They include the three branched-chain amino acids, which are the most important for building muscle. One of those, leucine, is the most powerful of all.

Animal proteins are considered "complete" because they contain all nine essential aminos in sufficient quantities to build new tissue. Your body can make complete proteins from incomplete sources eaten at various meals over the course of a day—rice and beans is the classic example—but it's not the easiest way to do things.

*Dietary Protein and Resistance Exercise* explains that a trained lifter will maximize protein synthesis with about 1.5 grams of leucine. (An untrained lifter may need as much as 2 grams to top out the protein response, although that's based on one small study.) The following chart shows the amount of leucine in foods most of us eat. Although some of the plant foods have generous portions of leucine, soy is the only vegetable protein with enough of the nine essential amino acids to build new tissue without combining with other foods.

| Food source | Serving size | Protein grams | Leucine grams |
|---|---|---|---|
| Almonds | ¼ cup | 6.6 | 0.5 |
| Beef (sirloin) | 4 oz. | 21 | 1.6 |
| Black beans | 1 cup | 15 | 1.2 |
| Chicken | ½ breast | 30 | 2.2 |
| Corn | 1 cup | 5 | 0.5 |
| **Cottage cheese** | **1 cup** | **28** | **2.9** |
| Eggs | 3 whole | 18 | 1.6 |
| Lentils | 1 cup | 16 | 1.3 |
| Milk, 2% | 2 cups | 16 | 1.6 |
| Mozzarella cheese | 3 oz. | 16 | 1.6 |
| Oats | ½ cup | 13 | 1.0 |
| Peanut butter | 2 Tbsp. | 8 | 0.7 |
| Pork loin | 5 oz. | 20 | 1.6 |
| Salmon | 4 oz. | 23 | 1.8 |
| **Soybeans** | **1 cup** | **29** | **2.3** |
| Whole-wheat bread | 2 slices | 5 | 0.4 |
| Wild rice | ½ cup | 11 | 0.8 |

*Source: Nutrition Almanac,* sixth edition.

## DO I NEED PROTEIN SUPPLEMENTS?

No.

## DO PROTEIN SUPPLEMENTS HELP?

I can't prove this, but I think the answer is yes. A lot of the research I cite in *Supercharged* (and the entire NROL series, for that matter) used protein supplements either as an independent variable—some people got it, some didn't—or to control the subjects' nutrition status to keep it from becoming a wild card.

Anecdotally, the most successful lifters all seem to use protein supplements. So do I, and so do Alwyn and his clients. The people I quote in this chapter, like Aragon and Phillips, certainly do. Most of Aragon's clients do. I'm not a supplement pusher, but I'd be doing you a disservice if I didn't tell you they probably help, and certainly can't hurt.

I would also recommend a post-workout protein shake for older lifters. A recent study at Purdue University compared the effects of a liquid meal replacement vs. a solid meal for a group of men and women in their early seventies. Those getting the liquid meal had higher amino acid concentrations in their blood both immediately and four hours afterward. It was a small study, and it didn't involve exercise, so there's only so much to read into it. But I don't think I'm going out on a limb to say that if you struggle to put on muscle, getting some protein in liquid form will ensure that your muscles have plenty to work with exactly when they need it.

## WHICH TYPE OF PROTEIN SUPPLEMENT IS BEST?

Most are made from milk proteins: whey and/or casein. The protein in a glass of milk is 80 percent casein and just 20 percent whey, but most supplements are entirely or mostly whey, usually in the form of whey isolate. A post-workout shake with 20 to 25 grams of whey isolate will contain 2 to 3 grams of leucine—plenty to max out protein synthesis. Whey is also the fastest-acting protein, which means it's the fastest to digest, reach your muscles, and then exit your system.

Casein is slower to digest, and for that reason is usually regarded as an inferior post-workout supplement. Curiously, several studies have shown that casein inhibits protein breakdown, which may mean it's a good choice for those who're mostly interested in weight loss. Someone who's doing hard workouts while cutting calories will probably lose some muscle. Casein may help stem the losses.

If you go back to the leucine chart, you'll see that I highlighted cottage cheese, the curds of which are predominantly casein. (The liquid is whey.) You'll see that it packs a lot of leucine in a single serving. If you aren't worried about how fast the protein reaches your muscles, cottage cheese may be the cheapest and best "supplement" you can buy.

I also highlighted soybeans—a complete protein with a generous portion of leucine. Until recently I was convinced that soy protein was a terrible choice for men. It contains phytoestrogens, which at minimum would give us cooties, and at worst would lower our testosterone levels. (At my age, I need all I can retain.) As a supplement, soy protein isolate has traditionally been considered the fourth-best choice for muscleheads, behind whey, casein, and egg protein. Which means it's in last place. If supplements were soccer teams in the English Premier League, soy would be relegated to a lower division.

So it's interesting to read in *Dietary Protein and Resistance Exercise* that soy isolate performs just as well as whey over six to twelve weeks of training and supplementation. That is, muscle gains were the same no matter which type of protein the lifters consumed after their workouts.

## SHOULD I ADD CREATINE?

I think it's a good idea if you want to increase muscle strength and size. We now have twenty years' worth of research showing it's safe for everyone and effective for most of us. Once your muscles are fully saturated—which should take about a month if you use 3 to 5 grams of creatine monohydrate per day—you can expect strength increases of about 5 to 15 percent. In my admittedly limited experience, these strength gains seem to come out of nowhere, and for the first couple of weeks after they kick in you'll feel like a superhero.

You should also see a pretty quick increase in muscle mass, perhaps as much as two to four pounds. Turning once more to *Dietary Protein and Resistance Exercise* (a $100 textbook that would've been a bargain at double the price), the process looks like this:

1. Creatine pulls water into muscle cells.
2. That leads to swollen cells, which put pressure on surrounding tissues.
3. This sends a signal to your satellite cells, which, thanks to their secret decoder rings, tells them it's okay to have intimate relations with your muscle fibers, impregnating them with extra nuclei.
4. Your muscles end up bigger and stronger, and I assume much happier at the cellular level.

(At least, I think that's what the book says. Steps 2 and 3 involve a long list of hormones, enzymes, and contractile tissues that I'd need an advanced degree to understand, so I kind of extrapolated the romantic subplot.)

Creatine also seems to deliver some surprising benefits that go beyond strength and hypertrophy. Because it increases the supply of energy in your cells (remember that creatine phosphate is a fuel source during short efforts requiring all-out strength and power), it also improves neural and cognitive performance. That is, you think a little faster and move a little better.

# Let's Get Small

EVERYONE KNOWS HOW TO GET BIGGER. Lift big, eat big, sleep big. But when it comes to body composition—carrying the most muscle with the least fat—we tear up the playbook every few years, and convince ourselves that what we used to believe couldn't possibly be true. The more extreme the new plan, the more likely we are to give it credibility.

When I started as a fitness writer in the early nineties, we just accepted that you needed to eat an extreme low-fat diet and do lots of long, slow cardio if you wanted to get exceptionally lean. That's what the competitive bodybuilders did, and whatever they do tends to filter down to the rest of us, through personal trainers and other fitness experts who act as intermediaries. Those of us who aspired to the muscular ideal assumed they must know what they're talking about.

Today's accepted wisdom is the opposite: We should eat extreme low-carb diets and get lean with high-intensity interval training. This circles back to the ideas of Vince Gironda, a bodybuilding guru of the pre-steroid era. (I used to drive past

Vince's Gym in North Hollywood on my way to work at Weider Publications. At the time I had no idea who "Vince" was.) He advocated drinking whole milk by the gallon and eating dozens of fertilized eggs. Other than the milk, it was a low-carb diet. His training programs emphasized density—getting lots of work done in a compressed amount of time—rather than length.

Where is this going? Five or ten years from now, will the cutting-edge trainers in the fitness industry be talking about low-fat diets again, along with long, slow cardio for fat loss? Will someone come up with a clever hybrid that mixes and matches everything in a new and unexpected way? Your guess is as good as mine. The one thing I *don't* expect is that we'll be advocating the same diet and training programs we advocate now.

Let's start the ruling there, and see if we can find some threads that connect seemingly opposed ideas about getting lean without sacrificing muscle.

## NEW RULE #21  •  Everything works better when you're strong.

Alwyn is a big advocate of metabolic resistance training—performing combinations of strength exercises in a way that spikes your heart rate and leaves you gasping for breath. He has his clients do the drills toward the end of workouts, and it works better than anything else to help them lose fat. Before that he tried everything from steady-pace cardio to all-out sprints.

The metabolic circuits are most effective in conjunction with a solid strength-training program. "Otherwise, it doesn't seem to work very well," he says. Nor does endurance training work on its own for most of the people who try it. For that matter, it's also really hard to get lean using strength training alone. It builds muscle, but for most people it doesn't burn enough calories, or create enough of a post-exercise metabolic boost, to help you get much leaner than you already are.

What does work, Alwyn says, is strength training + just about anything. He likes to use high-repetition strength exercises, mixing and matching push-ups, lunges, squats, and rows, for example. Others like to use traditional endurance training, done at a slow pace. Strength and power athletes like to push and drag weighted sleds, or carry heavy objects for short distances.

Alwyn can only guess at why these disparate fat-loss routines seem to work about equally well in conjunction with strength training, but not so well on their own. It probably comes down to a delicate balance between three variables:

1. Workout volume
2. Workout intensity
3. Workout recovery

Working your muscles to exhaustion with relatively heavy loads hits all three drivers of muscle growth: mechanical tension, muscle damage, and metabolic stress. High-intensity intervals would pile on extra metabolic stress, and possibly muscle damage as well, complicating your recovery from one workout to the next. That's why bodybuilders tend to do well with low-intensity cardio. It burns extra calories without making anything else worse. Alwyn also notes that any exercise a successful bodybuilder does will burn more calories than it will for someone with less muscle mass.

At another extreme you have powerlifting-type workouts, which use near-maximum weights to create tremendous mechanical tension and muscle damage. But the level of metabolic stress may be relatively low. So when powerlifters do what they call GPP—general physical preparation—they'll do hard, fast, sprint-type drills. Those produce a lot of metabolic stress with relatively little muscle damage, due to the fact that muscle loading occurs in the concentric part of the exercise, when they're pushing or pulling. Their muscles are rarely under high stress while lowering a weight or recovering from a movement.

The strength portions of Alwyn's *Supercharged* workouts have fewer sets and reps than the ones in the original *NROL*, but in return you have more total movement via mobility, core training, power training, and metabolic resistance training. So you're creating some muscle damage and metabolic stress in other parts of the workout, but not so much that you compromise your recovery. The net effect, Alwyn has found after crunching numbers from hundreds of clients and thousands of workouts, is faster and more dependable fat loss.

## NEW RULE #22 • There's no such thing as a fat-burning food.

Protein does wonderful things for our bodies, and if you don't already know that, you haven't been paying attention. But its effects are hardly magical. It takes some effort to manage a higher-protein diet, and it takes pure, hard work to use that protein to build muscle. That kind of work at least produces lasting results. Searching for a secret food that melts calories is a waste of time.

The converse, I reluctantly admit, is also true: There's no such thing as a food that automatically increases your body fat. There are certainly crap foods, and I've explained in some detail in the NROL series how those foods are engineered to make it hard to stop eating once you begin. But I have yet to see evidence that small amounts of any single food lead to fat gain in the absence of an overall caloric surplus.

Which brings us to this:

## NEW RULE #23  •  All calories matter, whether they're going in or coming out.

The links between exercise, food, and body weight are not linear. Gain a couple of pounds and your metabolism speeds up. It becomes your new normal, and if you want to gain additional weight (which some of the men reading this hope to achieve, bizarre as that sounds to most of the women), you have to find a way to eat slightly more. Same with initial weight loss. Cut some calories, and you'll lose some weight. Your body will then adjust your metabolism to compensate, and you'll need to find a new way to achieve a caloric imbalance and lose more weight. But no matter how complicated the math gets, the basic addition and subtraction of calories is still more important than anything else.

Five ways to subtract calories:

1. **Move more.** However you can, whenever you can. If nothing else, just get out of your chair more often.
2. **Cut the calories you won't miss.** Your body is too smart not to notice huge energy decreases—cutting 500 to 1,000 daily calories, for example. But if you measure your food and create small decreases in portion sizes, you can eat less without feeling worse.
3. **Eat more protein and less of everything else.** About 10 percent of the calories you burn each day come from the thermic effect of food (TEF). Protein has a much higher TEF than carbs or fat; as much as 25 percent of protein burns off during digestion. That compares to about 6 to 8 percent for carbs and 2 to 3 percent for fat.
4. **Burn more calories during your workouts.** You can do this via volume or intensity, and Alwyn's *Supercharged* workouts give you plenty of opportunity for both.
5. **Create metabolic stress in your workouts.** This should increase your metabolic rate in the hours following your workout. I can't say how substantial it is, or how long it lasts. It's going to vary from person to person based on your weight, nutri-

tion, and training status (more experienced lifters and athletes can probably generate more of an "afterburn" effect), even if both people do the exact same workout. But it has some effect, and helps explain why some programs work better than others.

## HOW TO LOSE FAT

Just a few short years ago, better body composition seemed so simple. Eat four to six medium-sized meals a day with more or less equal amounts of the three macronutrients (carbs, fat, protein), avoid fast food, work out hard and consistently, and the fat comes off. The more fat you have to lose, and the more stubbornly it hangs on, the more rigid you have to be about your meals and workouts. You'll probably have to shift to a higher-protein, lower-carb diet. Regular exercise outside the weight room will also help. But we're still talking about a relatively simple plan.

Then everything started to change. Some people advocated paleo-type diets, which reject decades of nutrition science in favor of a more interesting proposition: We'd all be better off if we ate foods that were the foundation of human diets before the invention of agriculture. That means lots of meat, fish, eggs, vegetables, and fruits, but no grains, dairy, or legumes—a category that includes beans, peas, peanuts and peanut butter, soybeans, and lentils.

Some people switched to a raw-foods diet, based on the idea that cooking destroys the most health-promoting enzymes and nutrients. Cooking also makes food easier to digest and use for energy, which is why people on raw-food diets tend to lose weight quickly and easily—their bodies simply can't make efficient use of the nutrients.

And lots of people, for lots of reasons, use intermittent fasting (IF), which turns upside down the idea that we're all best off eating a series of small meals at predictable times each day. Some IFers go for a long stretch each day without any food, skipping breakfast, lunch, dinner, or some combination. Others have a twenty-four-hour fast once a week.

What they all have in common is that many of the smartest people I know are the first to try them. They often become the most passionate advocates, in part, I suspect, because of the thrill of overturning conventional wisdom. The speculative nature of the diets becomes the biggest source of their appeal.

Eventually, as always happens in the fitness business, the first-movers compete to see who can go one step beyond everyone else. If lots of people are trying one complicated intervention, someone will come out in favor of doing multiple interven-

## The Power of an Extreme Diet

In *Scott Pilgrim vs. the World*, a vegan challenges Scott, the movie's hero, to a fight. Here's how Todd, the vegan, explains his diet: "I partake not of the meat, nor the breast milk, nor the ovum of any creature with a face."

The joke is that his vegan diet gives him physical and mental superpowers. When one of Scott's friends asks how not eating dairy made him psychic, Todd says, "Okay, you know how you only use 10 percent of your brain? That's because the other 90 percent is filled with curds and whey."

Another of Scott's friends scoffs, and Todd shoots her down with this: "Go ahead and get snippy, baby. If you knew the science, maybe I'd listen to a word you're saying."

It's funny because, at any given minute on any given day, somebody is saying exactly that to justify a nontraditional diet.

tions. We end up with people doing intermittent fasts on a raw-food version of the paleo diet, with workouts that are more grueling than the ones used by timid, well-fed enthusiasts like me. I don't know if it's a race to the top or the bottom. Whatever it is, it leaves those of us who're using garden-variety diets and workouts feeling like we're missing something. We begin to question whether the tried and true are truly tried, and actually true. Is it possible we've gotten everything wrong?

That's why, when I was assigned to write an article about the paleo diet for *Men's Health* magazine, I was happy to give it a shot. To be honest, I didn't expect it to work, for lots of reasons. The history buff in me objected to the simplified view of human evolution. There was never a time when all our ancestors ate the same things, or when we were so perfectly adapted to our environment that we stopped evolving. The environment changed, sometimes rapidly, and humans survived because we adapted to change itself. We could thrive on meat or plants, in hot or cold climates, as predators or prey. The fastest evolutionary adaptations in the past few thousand years are to dairy, grains, and other new foods introduced since the rise of agriculture and the domestication of animals for food.

I started in early January 2012. I never went 100 percent paleo (I stuck with my whole-grain cereal and milk for breakfast), but I mostly cut out grains for the rest of the day. In fact, I'm pretty sure I didn't have my first sandwich or slice of pizza until mid-May. To fill the gap, I ate more fruit the first few months of 2012 than I typically do in a year. It was inconvenient at times—try enjoying a family dinner of meatballs without spaghetti—but I did lose a few pounds, and I think most of it was fat.

These are my takeaway lessons, which I think apply to all fat-loss interventions, simple or complex:

## THE BEST FAT-LOSS DIET IS THE ONE YOU CAN LIVE WITH

Any diet that leaves you hungry will probably fail sooner or later. I suppose there's someone, somewhere who can go on for years with that empty-stomach feeling. I certainly can't. Your goal is to find a way to eat less without your body sensing an acute change in your normal calorie intake. That means you have to bias your diet toward foods that create more satiety, allowing you to go longer before you feel hungry again.

The satiety index is a scale created to put different foods into this context. It starts with white bread, which is given a score of 100. Anything under 100 is less satiating, and anything over 100 is probably more useful for weight control.

## HIGH SATIETY

| Food | Satiety Index |
|---|---|
| Apple | 197 |
| Baked beans | 168 |
| Banana | 118 |
| Beef | 176 |
| Bread, white | 100 |
| Bread, whole-grain | 157 |
| Doughnuts | 68 |
| Eggs | 150 |
| Ice cream | 96 |
| Pasta, white | 119 |
| Pasta, whole-wheat | 188 |
| Potato (baked) | 323 |
| Rice, brown | 132 |
| Rice, white | 138 |

*Source:* mendosa.com/satiety.htm; a version of this chart originally appeared in *The New Rules of Lifting for Abs,* page 217.

## THE BEST WEIGHT-MAINTENANCE DIET IS PROBABLY HIGH IN PROTEIN AND LOW IN CARBS

Among gym rats, I think this is a settled question, but for some reason it remains a subject of debate everywhere else. A fascinating study in the *Journal of the American Medical Association* may finally put it to rest. Researchers at Boston Children's Hospital started with a group of young adults who had just lost 10 to 15 percent of their initial body weight. They then cycled them through three different diets that had been calculated to give them the exact number of calories they needed to maintain their current weight. The diets were the usual suspects:

- High-carb, low-fat (60 percent carbs, 20 percent fat, 20 percent protein)
- Medium-carb, medium-fat (40 percent carbs, 40 percent fat, 20 percent protein)
- Very low carb, high-fat (10 percent carbs, 60 percent fat, 30 percent protein)

The low-fat diet used high-glycemic-index carbohydrates, which means those that digest the fastest, including grains, starchy vegetables, and fruits. The in-between diet used low-glycemic-index carbs, including slower-digesting legumes. The final diet was based on Atkins.

The participants went through the diets in random order, staying on each one for a month.

Here's the fascinating part: When participants were on Atkins, they burned about 300 more calories a day than they did on the low-fat diet. This is despite eating the same amount of food, in the same conditions. Just by eating different types of food, their metabolic processes shifted into a higher gear, which would make it easier to maintain their new, reduced weight. But the researchers also found that subjects had higher levels of cortisol, a stress hormone, when they were eating super-low carbs, and noted that it's nearly impossible for people in nonclinical settings to stay on a diet with just 10 percent carbs.

All in all, they recommended the in-between diet, the one with moderate levels of fat and slowly digesting carbs. I would think that most of us would do even better if we lowered the carbs and increased the protein to make each about 30 percent of your total calories. Of course that's just a guess, but it comes from many years of seeing people fail at the extremes but do well by tweaking diets to make them sustainable. There's a lot of ground between Atkins and Olive Garden.

## SUBSTRATES MATTER

Your body taps into two main energy substrates for fuel: fat and carbohydrate. The carbs you eat are converted to glucose during digestion, and then either burned or stored as glycogen. At any given time you have just a few grams of glucose in your bloodstream, and anywhere from 400 to 800 grams of glycogen stashed in your muscles and liver. At 4 calories per gram, you'd have between 1,600 and 3,200 calories of energy. Even if your body let you use all of it, it would barely keep you going for a day. But your body would never let you do that. It fights to defend your glycogen, and you get hungry as a bear when it sinks below your customary level.

Fat, on the other hand, offers a nearly unlimited supply of energy. Let's say you weigh 150 pounds, with 20 percent body fat. That gives you 30 pounds of fat, which is about 123,000 calories. Assuming you use a million calories in a year, isn't it mind-blowing to think that you're carrying more than 10 percent of them on your body right now?

Then again, you wouldn't actually want to use all of them, and if you starved yourself to the point that you used even half, your metabolism would punish you by slowing down dramatically. On top of that, your body would most likely tap into the one energy substrate you don't want to deplete: the protein in your muscles.

Therefore, you want to get your body to tap often and deeply into your fat stores, without slowing your metabolism or losing any muscle. Most paradigm-challenging diets aim to do exactly that, via different mechanisms. The paleo diet, for example, gives you plenty of protein, with fairly low carbohydrates. A low-carb diet encourages your body to use more fat for energy throughout the day, with the goal of preserving the glycogen stored in your muscles and liver.

Vegetarian and raw-foods diets, on the other hand, are higher in carbs, but push your body to use the energy in an inefficient way. More of the food ends up excreted, which means less is available for your body to burn.

Finally, a person who's fasting has to tap into fat stores simply because there's nothing else for the body to use for energy, other than the protein in your muscles. You can easily replace that by lifting and eating lots of protein afterward.

## ANY SET OF RULES THAT MAKES YOU THINK BEFORE EATING WILL PROBABLY HELP

None of us wants to overeat, but too often we can't help ourselves. We eat if everyone else is eating. Or if we're alone. Or if we're upset. Or if we're in a good mood. If mindless or emotion-triggered eating leads to an energy surplus, it seems logical that stopping to think before you eat is the path to an energy deficit. Any diet that gives you a firm set of rules—this is okay, that isn't—should help you manage calories.

The rules still have to make sense, and they still have to allow enough food to avoid the kind of intense hunger that will derail any diet. Most important, they have to leave you with enough energy to do Alwyn's workouts, the subject of the rest of the book.

# PART 3

# THE SYSTEM

# How the Workouts Work

ALWYN'S *SUPERCHARGED* SYSTEM has two unique components:

## You choose your own exercises from the menus we provide

The workouts, which you'll find starting in Chapter 19, are presented as templates. The template tells you which movement pattern to do, along with the number of sets and repetitions. Each movement pattern has its own chapter in which we show you the exercise choices, ranked from Level 1 to Level 5. Where possible I've included notes about which exercises and variations work best for different goals and different types of programs. If you're lifting for the first time, you can simply start with Level 1 exercises for each movement pattern, and then advance to higher-level exercises when you're ready.

## You choose your own progression through a series of ten programs

Readers of the original *NROL* are familiar with the idea of navigating their way through a series of programs (just as readers of *NROL for Life* are used to selecting their own exercises).

Each program includes two total-body workouts, labeled Workout A and Workout B. You'll never do A and B on the same day. Nor do you want to do A and B on consecutive days. Three workouts a week (Monday/Wednesday/Friday, for example, or Tuesday/Thursday/Saturday) is a good target for most of us, but if you're too busy, or your body needs longer to recover between workouts, then two is fine. One is too few to see results, and four is too many.

Here's what a month of training will look like if you follow the classic Monday-Wednesday-Friday workout schedule:

|  | Monday | Tuesday | Wednesday | Thursday | Friday | Saturday | Sunday |
|---|---|---|---|---|---|---|---|
| **Week 1** | Workout A | off | Workout B | off | Workout A | off | off |
| **Week 2** | Workout B | off | Workout A | off | Workout B | off | off |
| **Week 3** | Workout A | off | Workout B | off | Workout A | off | off |
| **Week 4** | Workout B | off | Workout A | off | Workout B | off | off |

You can do other types of exercise on the days you don't lift. In fact, we encourage it, as you'll see in Chapter 23. But you'll need at least two days—48 hours—between *Supercharged* workouts. You'll alternate between these workouts until you've completed the program. (What "completed" means will be slightly different for each one; you'll see what I mean when you get to those chapters.) Then you'll move on to the next program.

## THE PROGRAMS

Here's a quick overview of the ten programs:

### Basic Training I, II, III, and IV

In the original *NROL* the first program was called Break-In; it was followed by Fat Loss I, II, and III. We regretted these labels from the very beginning, and wanted a do-over. The biggest problem is the labels themselves. Experienced lifters didn't want to start with a Break-In program, and readers most interested in building muscle size and strength didn't want to start with programs labeled Fat Loss.

With *Supercharged* we call the first four programs Basic Training because we want to emphasize the importance of starting at the beginning. Just don't confuse "basic" with "entry-level." Alwyn and his trainers certainly use them with beginners, but Alwyn has also used these templates in the programs he's written for famous, highly paid professional athletes. These are men and women whose living depends on being in top condition. Not one has ever stopped in the middle and said to his trainer, "Hey, isn't this a beginner workout?"

Basic Training works for all types of lifters because you select your own exercises, and make them as hard as you want them to be. If a workout seems too easy, it's because you need to choose more challenging exercises, or heavier weights, or perhaps a faster pace.

So you may wonder: Why not just make up your own workouts from scratch? Fair question, with a simple answer: Your own workouts will probably stink. You'll do your favorite exercises first. You'll skimp on core training, unless you happen to like it, in which case you may do more than you need. You'll avoid anything you don't enjoy, even if it means skipping entire movement patterns. You might improve in whatever it is you're most concerned with—more of this, less of that—but you'll probably go backward in other areas. You could end up lean but weak, strong but fat, bigger but less athletic.

Or, perhaps, you'll write great programs for yourself. Kudos if you can. I've been working out since 1970, writing about fitness since 1992, and certified as a trainer since 1997. And I still create all the problems I just described when I make up my own programs.

## Hypertrophy I, II, and III

These will look familiar to readers of the original *NROL*. They're based on the same system of undulating periodization. That is, you'll alternate workouts in which you work with heavy, medium, and light loads. But the program templates—the mix of exercises in each workout—are more like the plans in *NROL for Life*. Instead of doing all your upper-body training in Workout A and all the lower-body exercises in Workout B, you'll do total-body workouts each time.

## Strength & Power I, II, and III

These programs are more complex than Basic Training and Hypertrophy. In addition to the A and B workouts, you also have C and D in the final two programs. Each focuses on developing strength and power in one movement pattern: squat, push (usually the bench press), hinge (usually a deadlift variation), and pull (either a chin-up or row). In addition, the configuration of sets and reps differs quite a bit for Strength I, II, and III. I'll explain in detail in Chapter 21.

# ELEMENTS OF THE WORKOUTS

Each workout of each program includes all or most of these elements, usually in this order.

### 1. RAMP (Chapter 17)

The acronym stands for *Range of motion, Activation of muscles,* and *Movement Preparation.* Or you can just call it the warm-up. This part of the workout usually takes about 10 minutes—slightly more if all the exercises are new to you, slightly less as you get familiar with them. You won't choose your own RAMP exercises, unless you decide to tweak Alwyn's selection. I recommend at least trying it the way it's shown in Chapter 17 so you get the idea of how Alwyn wants you to prepare for these workouts.

### 2. Core Training (Chapter 14)

The core, in our definition, includes all the muscles that attach to and help stabilize the lower back and pelvis, keeping it in a safe, neutral position. Alwyn has two major categories of core exercises: *stabilization,* in which you're holding a fixed position for timed sets, and *dynamic stabilization,* in which you're moving one or more limbs while maintaining a stable core.

### 3. Combination and Power Exercises (Chapter 15)

Power exercises are a crucial component in the four Basic Training programs. Alwyn doesn't include them in the Hypertrophy and Strength & Power programs because, as I noted earlier, you'll cover the territory by using heavier weights and including some high-speed metabolic drills.

Combination exercises include two distinct movement patterns—a squat and a press, for example, or a deadlift and row. They challenge your balance and coordination along with your core stability. But mostly they take more energy to perform, increasing the metabolic cost of the workout.

### 4. Strength Training

You'll use these movement patterns in each program:

- Squat (Chapter 8)
- Hinge (Chapter 9)

- Push (Chapter 10)
- Pull (Chapter 11)
- Lunge (Chapter 12)
- Single-Leg Stance (Chapter 13)

There are four lower-body movement patterns, and just two for the upper body. Alwyn divides the lower-body movements so you do two of them in Workout A and the other two in B. You might have a squat and lunge in A, followed by a hinge (aka deadlift) and single-leg-stance exercise in B.

You'll do a push and pull each workout. Most often, you want to choose a vertical push and pull one workout and a horizontal push and pull in the other. In this case, "horizontal" describes your posture if you were doing the exercise from an upright posture. But when you're working with free weights, gravity requires you to lift them vertically. Thus, you have to put your body in a horizontal posture to execute a "horizontal" push or pull. The best-known examples are the push-up and bent-over row, although you can also do standing presses and rows with resistance bands or a cable machine. The lat pulldown and chin-up are vertical pulls, while the shoulder press (along with some push-up variations you'll see in Chapter 10) is a vertical push.

### 5. Metabolic Training (Chapter 16)

This a grab-bag category that can include lots of exercises and methods, depending on the program and your goals at the time:

- **Intervals** are timed exercises. You'll do them in the first three Basic Training programs. The intervals in Basic Training I use a work-rest ratio of 1 to 2: 1 minute of work, followed by 2 minutes of rest. Then you'll switch to shorter, faster-paced intervals: 30 seconds on, 60 seconds off. In Basic Training III you'll challenge yourself with a 1 to 1 ratio: 30 seconds on, 30 seconds off.
- **Complexes** are groups of exercises performed consecutively without rest, using the same weight. A classic example is a barbell complex in which you do several reps of Romanian deadlifts, cleans (an exercise in which you pull from your thighs to the top of your shoulders), and front squats or shoulder presses, all without setting down the bar. If your goal is 6 reps, for example, you do 6 of one exercise, then the next, then the last. Then you set the bar down, rest, and do it a few more times.
- **Free Zone** includes single or paired exercises to supplement the strength program.

You can emphasize fat loss by doing a lot of repetitions of several exercises, or focus on muscle by doing traditional supersets (two exercises for opposing muscle groups, with little or no rest in between) within a defined amount of time. You can superset exercises for your chest and back, for example, or even for biceps and triceps.

### 6. Recovery (Chapter 17)

Before you leave the gym, you'll begin preparing your body for the next workout by stretching and/or using a foam roller to work the kinks out of your muscles.

## HOW TO CHOOSE THE RIGHT EXERCISES FOR YOU

In *NROL for Life* we compared exercise selection to a Chinese menu. But instead of picking a soup, a meat, a vegetable, a sauce, and rice or noodles, you'll be picking a squat, hinge, lunge, and single-leg-stance exercise for each program, along with two pushes and two pulls for each program (one of each for the A and B workouts, as noted above). In addition, you'll need to select exercises for core, power, and metabolic training.

I know it sounds daunting. But it's easier than you think. For each movement pattern I'll give you some guidelines to decide where to start, along with some notes suggesting exercises for specific types of workouts and goals. Some exercises lend themselves to high repetitions, but aren't great choices when you're using heavy weights for low reps. Exercises that require the most balance and coordination are often best for fat loss, while the ones that give you the most solid base of support (barbell squats and deadlifts, for example) are almost always the best choices for hypertrophy and strength development.

These are the rules you must follow:

### 1. Stay true to the category.

Alwyn classifies exercises in a slightly different way from other trainers and coaches, and in some cases the classifications are different from our previous books. The biggest change from *NROL* and *NROL for Women* is that "lunge" and "single-leg stance" are now separate categories, and the latter now includes some exercises that were once in the hinge/deadlift category. The distinctions aren't always intuitive. But they're important for achieving balanced strength and muscle quality.

## 2. When in doubt, start with the easiest exercise you can use.

Let's say you're about to start with Basic Training I, which calls for 1 to 2 sets of 15 reps for each exercise. You know you need to choose two pulling exercises, one each for Workout A and Workout B. Leaving out all the options and alternatives for now, these are the basic choices for each level:

*Level 1:* Standing cable row

*Level 2:* Kneeling lat pulldown

*Level 3:* Dumbbell bent-over row

*Level 4:* Inverted or suspended row (pulling yourself up to a low bar, like a push-up in reverse)

*Level 5:* Chin-up or pull-up

You want one pull to be horizontal and one to be vertical. Most trainers in most gyms would start you with two seated exercises: the seated cable row, and the seated lat pulldown. But Alwyn doesn't want you to sit for anything. So, instead, you'll do the standing cable row (Level 1) in one workout, and the kneeling lat pulldown (Level 2) in the other. They require more attention to posture and form than the seated versions, but they're still simple exercises. More important, they're good exercises for just about any lifter . . . at least for a while.

On the standing row, you're limited by your ability to maintain your posture while pulling increasingly heavy weights to your torso. Sooner or later you'll need to move on to dumbbell rows, the Level 3 exercise, where you're only limited by the amount of weight you have available. (Me, I've never gotten close to maxing out my gym's dumbbells.)

The kneeling pulldown and its variations can keep you busy longer, but you still want to move on to more advanced exercises when you can. Inverted rows, the Level 4 exercise, are sort of in between vertical and horizontal pulls, and they're a great exercise to work on until you're strong enough to do chin-ups, the Level 5 exercise. (If you're strong enough to do chin-ups right away, for sets of 15 reps, you're golden. You can do any pulling exercise you want for any program in the book.)

### 3. When possible, change exercises when you change programs.

This is especially important with the four Basic Training programs. If you can, work your way through four different levels of each movement pattern. If you can't, at least switch to a different variation for the same level. (We give you a couple of options for most levels in most movement patterns.)

This will be harder to do in the Hypertrophy and Strength & Power programs. Most of us will probably use the same squat, deadlift, bench press, and row or chin-up for all the workouts that call for heavy weights. Alwyn hits you with a lot of different combinations of sets and reps, so the workouts will give you plenty of new challenges even with the same exercises. But you still want to change things up when the opportunity arises, for two big reasons:

- You don't want your body to do the exercise with too much efficiency; a little unfamiliarity goes a long way when it comes to creating metabolic stress, which is important for both fat loss and muscle development.
- You don't want to move your joints through the exact same range of motion for months on end until there's no other option. Workouts that call for higher repetitions are the perfect time to mix things up.

## HOW TO USE THE TEN PROGRAMS

Almost everyone who reads and uses *Supercharged* should start at the beginning, with Basic Training I, followed by Basic Training II, III, and IV. What you do next will depend on your success with Basic Training, as well as your goals. Most will want to move on to Hypertrophy I, II, and III. But some, as I'll explain in a moment, will get better results by repeating Basic Training I through IV.

The decision-making process starts with an honest assessment of your history and skill as a lifter. The following categories are meant to be descriptive, not demeaning, insulting, accusing. You don't know where to go until you understand where you are now, and how you got there.

### Beginner

If you've never lifted before, or haven't lifted in years, your decision is easy. You know you're a beginner, and any objective assessment would confirm it. But most of the people who *don't* consider themselves beginners are, in the context of Alwyn's programs, just that. This applies to almost everyone you see in a health club, including some who've been lifting for years.

See if you recognize yourself or anyone you know in the following categories.

## The Machinist

You've been going to your favorite health club for years, but you've never gotten past the machines and tried a workout based on barbells and dumbbells. Have you gotten stronger? Probably. Are your muscles bigger? I sure hope so. Is your physique impressive, in a seventy-fifth-percentile kind of way, adjusted for age, gender, and profession? It's entirely possible.

But are you a lifter? Absolutely not. If you don't know how to squat and deadlift with a barbell, or do lunges with some form of resistance, or knock out push-ups with the form you see in Chapter 10, or complete at least one good chin-up with your full body weight, you need to start at the beginning.

## The Dabbler

You've done some of everything: machines, barbells, dumbbells, endurance training, Spinning, boot camps, yoga. Maybe you've swung a kettlebell or two. You're willing to try anything, which will come in handy when you tackle Alwyn's programs. Even better, you probably have a nice base of muscular endurance and overall conditioning. That's terrific, because getting through these workouts will be a challenge for those who don't yet have those qualities.

Thing is, you've never done enough lifting to develop skill, strength, power, and the physiological transformations that go along with them. Your muscles are relatively small, and your connective tissues don't have the thickness and tensile strength they'll need to tackle the Hypertrophy and Strength & Power programs. The Basic Training programs may look easy on paper. But if they're easy to execute, as I've said many times already, you're doing them wrong.

## The Lightweight

You're convinced of one or more of the following:

(a) Heavy weights will break you.

(b) Heavy weights are for people who look like they lift heavy weights.

(c) Heavy weights will make you look like someone who lifts heavy weights, and it's not a look you aspire to.

(d) Heavy weights are hard to lift.

Let's take them in order:

You may never get around to lifting truly heavy weights. In fact, most of us don't. Weights that appear heavy when you're starting out are much less intimidating by the time you're finally strong enough to lift them. By then, of course, you know those weights won't break you, and you're amazed you were ever afraid of them.

Every time I go to the gym I see women (and some men) using weights that are clearly much lighter than they could handle for what I assume is their primary goal: a leaner, stronger, better-looking physique. How do I know the weights are light? The women can lift them repeatedly without any obvious effort, and stop well short of muscular exhaustion, signs of which include:

- a change in rep speed
- a shift in posture
- shaking arms or legs
- ragged breath
- sweat

Moving on:

Nobody achieves the look of a bodybuilder or powerlifter by accident. We all have a genetically determined shape, but how we use that shape is up to us. While anyone can manipulate diet to get somewhat leaner or thicker, it takes years of hard work to look like a strength athlete. Even when you're born with an aptitude for it. Putting in the work may have been an obvious choice for them, but it was a choice nonetheless.

Finally, yes, heavy weights are hard to lift. That's the entire point. It's not supposed to be easy.

## The Specialist

You're a runner. Or a yogi. Or a Zumba teacher. Or a boot camp queen. Or an aspiring bodybuilder who knows three dozen variations on the biceps curl, and uses half of them in any given week. It doesn't really matter what you've specialized in. The key is what you *haven't* done: a relatively simple program of progressive resistance with the goal of improving lifting skill and overall muscular fitness.

If you haven't done it, your body hasn't yet adapted to it. That means you'll see results from Basic Training that you didn't think were possible for an "advanced" athlete like yourself.

## The Used-to-Be

Here are some of the things I used to be:

- baseball player (until age twelve, and then again for one season in my early fifties)
- high school football player
- stockman (loading and unloading trucks at WalMart)
- lifeguard
- day laborer
- waiter and bartender

I couldn't do any of those things today, not without weeks of training (or months, if I wanted to get back on the lifeguard stand). I mean, if I had to, I could show up for a job unloading trucks or waiting tables, and probably get through my first day. But it would be a while before I could work a full shift without a handful of ibuprofen.

Today I'm a lifter. That's it. I'm not even a strong lifter. If I wanted to tackle a powerlifting or Olympic weightlifting program, I'd have to start at the beginner level. Same with an advanced bodybuilding program, or CrossFit, or Pilates, or anything else my body isn't prepared to do. What I'm prepared to do is the type of training in *Supercharged*.

And you? It doesn't matter what you used to do. It doesn't matter what you assume you can do, based on what you once did. What matters is what you can do *today*. If that doesn't include regular, progressive training with barbells and dumbbells, using relatively heavy weights on basic exercises like deadlifts and squats, then you need to

## Your Supercharged Plan

For each Basic Training program, you want to do workouts A and B six times each before moving on to the next program. That's twelve total workouts, which should take you about a month to complete, assuming that you work out three times a week. It will take you four months to complete Basic Training I through IV if you go straight through without interruption.

start at the beginning. You need to re-master the exercises and re-establish your base of muscular fitness.

## Intermediate

Upon finishing the four Basic Training programs, most of you will probably meet my description of an intermediate-level lifter:

- You can do free-weight and/or body-weight exercises in all the basic movement patterns with good form.
- You have mastered Levels 1, 2, and 3 of most, if not all, categories.
- You saw steady improvements in strength in every exercise you performed in Basic Training I through IV.
- Your body has changed in measurable ways: your waist is smaller, while your arms and thighs are more muscular.
- Your clothes fit differently.
- While each workout is still hard, it's hard in a good way. You can get through it with a level of skill, confidence, and effort that is noticeably better than when you started.

Does that mean you're ready for the Hypertrophy programs? Not necessarily. If you were still making progress on each stage of Basic Training before moving on to the next, you *may* want to repeat those four stages before tackling Hypertrophy I, II, and III. This is especially important if your main goal is fat loss, and you've seen good results from your first time through Basic Training.

Use more advanced exercises, or the same exercises with heavier weights and higher volume. That is, if Alwyn's template calls for two or three sets, and you did two sets the first time, do three now.

Do the A and B workouts three or four times each before moving on to the next program. Your performance is key. If the third time you do A and B is no better than the second time, it's time to move on to the next program. If the third is better, do A and B a fourth and final time.

Now let's talk about some types of lifters who don't meet any of the descriptions in the Beginner section. Each will have slightly different needs and a slightly different strategy.

## The NROL Veteran

If you've completed the program in *NROL for Life*, start *Supercharged* with Basic Training IV and then move on to Hypertrophy. The first three Basic Training programs are similar to those in *Life*, and you've probably gotten what you need out of them.

If you've recently completed the program in *NROL*, *NROL for Women*, and/or *NROL for Abs*, but not *Life*, start with Basic Training I, but do A and B four times each before moving on to Basic Training II.

## The Lifter Who Doesn't Look Like a Lifter

I know how it feels to hear, "Wait, you work out?" Once, in my mid-thirties, I made the mistake of telling an older, know-it-all guy in the gym that I'd been working out for twenty-plus years. He gave me the look you'd give a homeless person who said he was panhandling to pay for his time-share in South Beach. The old guy in my gym didn't know shit, but he *looked* like a lifter. I may have known more than him (even though I still had a lot to learn); it didn't matter because I looked, at best, like a Dabbler.

The question you have to answer: *Why* don't you look like a lifter?

### YOU'RE STRONG BUT OVERWEIGHT

Start with Basic Training, and do the A and B workouts in every program four times each. It's possible that, in pursuit of size and strength, you've neglected higher-rep, higher-volume training. Shoot for maximum volume, and *crush* these workouts.

### YOU'RE BORED

You need a boot in the buttocks, and Alwyn's Basic Training programs will provide it. Follow the plan described for "strong but overweight."

### YOU HAVE COCKTAIL-PARTY AMBITIONS WITH KEGGER GENETICS

Through no fault of your own, your body resists muscle gain. (Been there!) Even worse, it may cling stubbornly to every ounce of lipid it can generate. Heavy weights are your ticket out of genetic purgatory. Start with Hypertrophy I, II, and III, and then go on to the Strength & Power programs. When you're finished with those, you can circle back and tear through Basic Training for a fat-loss stimulus.

**YOU'RE GOOD, YOU LOOK GOOD, AND EVERYONE KNOWS YOU'RE GOOD**

I'm jealous, but okay: Follow the same plan as "kegger genetics," knowing you'll get better results than your genetically disadvantaged peers.

## REQUIRED AND RECOMMENDED EQUIPMENT

Based on my e-mails, I'm going to guess that NROL readers split about fifty-fifty between those who work out in commercial health clubs and those who either work out at home or in small, poorly equipped facilities. That means a substantial percentage will get pissed off while reading this section. So I'll start by throwing a bone to some of the equipment-challenged: The less advanced you are, the more you can get done with limited tools. But everyone who reads this is still going to need a range of dumbbells, some bands, something solid to use as an anchor for the bands (you can loop them around a pillar or joist, for example), and some combination of a bench, box, and/or steps that are sturdy enough to hold your weight. It's not ideal, but it's possible to train with that bare-bones setup.

That won't work for most *Supercharged* readers, and I don't think you'd want it to work. You'd quickly max out your weights, and you'd get bored with your limited options.

The great thing about workout equipment is that you only have to buy it once. There's no membership fee to use it, beyond your mortgage or rent payments. It doesn't wear out, spoil, or expire. It doesn't even collect dust if you use it often enough. You can share it, sell it, pass it down to your heirs.

Now let's take a look at what you need, and what many of you will want. Unless otherwise specified, everything I mention here is available from Perform Better (performbetter.com).

### Dumbbells

You have two good options and one that's less good. First the good:

With fixed-weight dumbbells, you can start with 1-pound Barbie weights at Kmart and go all the way up to 150-pounders from York Barbell (yorkbarbell.com). Or you can get an adjustable dumbbell set; you can find PowerBlock and Bowflex sets that go from 5 to 50 pounds, and take up less floor space than a coffee table. If you have $1,300 to spend, PowerBlock also makes a deluxe set that goes up to 90 pounds, which is as much weight as most of us, male or female, would ever need to use for the dumbbell exercises in Alwyn's workouts.

The less good but still viable option is dumbbell handles and free weights. I grew up using these, and they're a royal pain to adjust, especially if you're doing multiple exercises in a compressed amount of time. There are two basic types: standard (1-inch-thick bar) and Olympic (2 inches thick where the weights slide on; 1 inch thick where you hold the bar). I've never seen or used the Olympic-type dumbbells, so I have no idea if they're worth buying. (At $40 per handle, they're pricey.) With the standard type, you're limited by suboptimal collars. Women will have trouble using pinch-grip collars; if they're any good, you'll need a lot of hand strength to get them on and off the bar. Spin-lock collars, in my experience, don't stay spun, so the weights are often in danger of falling off. Cast-iron collars with screw-on fasteners are the best for safety but the worst for convenience.

## Barbell and weight plates

As with dumbbells, you have a choice of a standard or Olympic bar. My older brother and I started out with a standard bar, part of a 110-pound set. The bar usually weighs 10 pounds, and barely holds the 95 pounds of plates that come with it. (The other 5 pounds are dumbbell handles and collars.) It's fine for those just starting out. You can buy additional standard plates (including 25-pounders) when you outgrow the starter set.

But for serious lifting, nothing beats an Olympic barbell set. The bar is 7 feet long and 45 pounds, and most sets I've seen for sale online come with 255 pounds in weights, for a total of 300 pounds. Women may prefer a smaller, lighter Olympic bar. You can find bars that are 5 or 6 feet long, and 35 pounds or less. (We used a 6-foot bar in some of the photos you'll see in the next few chapters, just because it was easier to fit the shorter bar into the frame.) It's more expensive, since you'll have to buy the bar and weights separately.

Also keep in mind that weight plates on their own can be useful training tools. They can provide a platform when you need to elevate your feet an inch or two, and they're a good substitute for dumbbells on some squat and lunge variations.

## Squat rack with chin-up bar

A good squat rack serves four purposes:

1. You can do front or back squats with the Olympic bar set up at shoulder height.
2. You can do inverted rows or elevated push-ups with the bar set at waist height or below.

3. You can do chin-ups and pull-ups from a fixed bar at the top.

4. You can attach bands or a suspension trainer (see below) to the chin-up bar, or attach bands to the vertical supports at any height you choose.

It takes up a lot of room. The footprint is about 20 square feet; you'll need a little more than 7 feet of clearance at the top and at least 2 feet on each side of the rack—about 8 to 9 feet altogether. But you can't beat the versatility. On top of giving you a place to do just about all the free-weight and body-weight exercises in *Supercharged*, you can choose a higher-end squat rack with an adjustable cable pulley for rows and pulldowns, with or without a selectorized weight stack (you use a pin to select the weight you want). A commercial-grade rack might also come with bars on the sides to store your weight plates when you aren't using them.

## Cable machine, bands, tubing

The cable setup I just described takes away the need for bands or tubing for your home gym. And just about any gym, private or commercial, will have at least one cable machine. But if you train at home, and don't have a cable system, you'll need bands or tubing to perform some of the exercises in Alwyn's program. (Bands are usually loops of rubber, at various thicknesses. Tubing is the same thing, only instead of a loop it has handles on the ends.) You have a huge range of options, from heavy-duty Superbands (the ones I use, and the ones you'll find in gyms like Alwyn's) to lighter Thera-Bands. Trainers like Gray Cook and Juan Carlos Santana have their own brands of bands. Then there are minibands, which are useful for injury rehab and for sport-specific training.

If you're interested, take some time to check out the options. You can find packages of bands and attachments, and countless single-band options. Start with the articles and videos at Perform Better. I also recommend Dave Schmitz's site, resistancebandtraining.com. Alwyn can probably show you dozens, if not hundreds, of band exercises, but Dave is the only trainer I know who *evangelizes* for them.

## Bench, box, steps

Most of us like to have a traditional weight bench, preferably one that inclines. It allows you to do bench presses, push-ups with your hands or feet elevated, and step-ups. You also want boxes or steps at various heights for the single-leg-stance exercises and some of the lunge and hinge variations. A set of aerobics steps should do the job. Really, anything that's flat and supports your body weight is fine.

### Suspension trainer

When Alwyn and I wrote *NROL for Abs*, which came out in early 2011, we mentioned that the best-known suspension system, the TRX, was "expensive" at $150. Today the TRX Pro Pack is closer to $200. But I've tried several others, including the $100 Jungle Gym XT, and haven't yet found one I like better.

Whichever one you pick, you'll be happy with the investment. It multiplies your options for core and body-weight exercises, and there are always new ones to learn— many of which, I admit, kick my ass before I run out of fingers counting the reps. (Check out trxtraining.com for the latest.)

All you need is an overhead attachment point, usually a chin-up bar. A ceiling joist or even a tree limb can also work.

### Foam roller

These $10 foam cylinders, 6 inches in diameter, went from novelty to necessity almost overnight. A few minutes of rolling before, after, or in between workouts will help you work out the adhesions and trigger points that all lifters accumulate.

### Kettlebells

I wouldn't say kettlebells are a necessity, but they sure make a workout more fun and interesting, especially for metabolic training. Men should get at least a 25- or 30-pound kettlebell to use for swings (shown on page 219), while women want at least a 15-pounder. As with bands and suspension trainers, your options just keep growing—more products, more exercises. I recommend starting with the articles and videos at Perform Better; also check out Steve Cotter's advice and tutorials at ikff.net.

### Also consider . . .

- A good Swiss ball gives you lots of options for core training. You can buy one anywhere. If you have a TRX, you may find, as Alwyn has, that you don't really need a Swiss ball. Both provide an unstable platform, but the TRX is more versatile.
- You'll need some kind of timer (I use the one on my iPhone) or clock for core and metabolic training.
- Alwyn and I are big fans of Valslides, which are $35 sliding discs you can use for a variety of core exercises.

# Squat

I USED TO WRITE SENTENCES like this: "The human body has more than 600 muscles, and the squat uses more than 250 of them." Now I like to quote Thomas Myers, author of *Anatomy Trains*, who believes the human body has one muscle with more than 600 compartments, separated by intricate bands, strands, and layers of connective tissues. Just about all of them come into play when you squat with a heavy weight.

Your hands, arms, and shoulders hold, balance, and support the weight. The muscles in your neck are on full alert, and the tension in your facial muscles twists your features until your driver's license photo starts to look flattering. Everything in your torso tightens up to provide stability to your spine and pelvis. The muscles in your hips and thighs provide the force to lift your body and the weight out of the bottom position, while your foot and lower-leg muscles are your body's first responders any time you're upright—especially when you're both upright and moving something heavy.

Your body can employ any number of strategies to get up and down in a squat. Some of us do better with a shoulder-width stance and toes pointed more or less straight ahead. Others squat with their heels closer together and toes pointed out.

Powerlifters squat with an extremely wide stance, which gives them more lift from muscles in the inner thighs and also activates muscles on the outside of the hips that help support the spine when it's under heavy loads. Some of us lean forward more than others.

What truly matters:

- You start the movement by pushing your hips backward, as if you're going to sit down on something.
- If you're squatting with a barbell, the bar is directly over the middle of your feet at the top and bottom of the movement, and all points in between. If you aren't using a barbell, your shoulders will be over your feet.
- Your feet are flat on the floor throughout the movement. If your heels come off the floor, you need to work on the mobility in your ankles. (If your toes come off the floor, you understand why alcohol and strength training don't mix.)

<u>LEVEL 1</u>

## ✳ Body-weight squat

**BEST FOR:** beginners only. If you can do 15 body-weight squats—I recommend testing yourself before your first workout—there's no reason to start with this one. But if you can't, stay at Level 1 until you can do 2 sets of 15, or until you finish Basic Training I, whichever comes first.

**GET READY**

- Stand with your feet shoulder-width apart, toes pointed forward or angled out slightly, and your arms straight out in front of you.

**MOVE**

- Push your hips straight back and descend until the tops of your thighs are parallel to the floor, with your knees directly over your toes.
- Rise back up to the starting position.

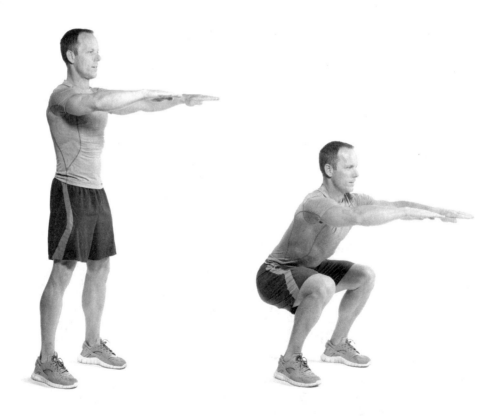

## LEVEL 2

### ✳ Goblet squat

**BEST FOR:** high-repetition sets in Basic Training. It's a great way to learn the squat movement pattern, and one that I hadn't yet heard of when Alwyn and I wrote the original *NROL*. We didn't include it in the series until *NROL for Life*. In just a few years it's gone from "remind me what that is again?" to a workout staple. The only drawback is that your hip strength will increase faster than your ability to hold a suitably heavy weight in front of your chest.

**GET READY**

- Grab a dumbbell or weight plate and hold it with both hands against your chest, just below your chin.
- Stand with your feet shoulder-width apart, with your toes pointed forward or angled out slightly.

**MOVE**

- Push your hips straight back and descend until the tops of your thighs are parallel to the floor.
- Rise back up to the starting position.

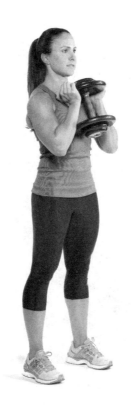
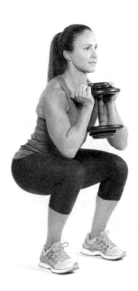

## Options

You can do a goblet squat with anything—dumbbell, weight plate, kettlebell (holding either the sides of the handle or the belly with both hands), medicine ball, or as strength coach Dan John (who popularized it) suggests, a big rock. It all works.

## Wimpus Interruptus

While I was writing this chapter, I watched a young, apparently healthy guy do a set of dumbbell shoulder presses with 25 pounds in each hand, then set one of the weights down and do a set of goblet squats using a single 25-pound dumbbell. I'd estimate it was less than half the weight he could've handled. Unless you're a novice or recovering from an injury, you want to be aggressive with exercises like squats and deadlifts. The muscles in your hips and thighs—gluteus maximus, hamstrings, quadriceps—are the biggest and strongest you have. When you get to a point where you can't hold a weight heavy enough to challenge those muscles, even on higher-rep sets, then you're finished with the goblet squat, and it's time to move on to a higher-level squat variation.

### LEVEL 2.5

## ✳ Kettlebell rack-position squat

**BEST FOR:** any program in Basic Training or Hypertrophy, any rep range. You're only limited by the pairs of kettlebells you have access to.

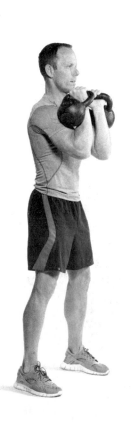

**GET READY**
- Grab a pair of kettlebells and hold them in the "rack" position—hands together near your chin, elbows pulled in, weights resting on the outside of your forearms and upper arms.
- Stand with your feet shoulder-width apart, with your toes pointed forward or angled out slightly.

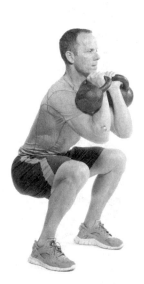

**MOVE**
- Push your hips straight back and descend until the tops of your thighs are parallel to the floor.
- Rise to the starting position.

SUPERCHARGE IT!

## ✴ Kettlebell offset rack-position squat

Hold a single kettlebell in the rack position. Do an equal number of reps with the weight on each side. If you're doing high-repetition sets, switch sides halfway through the set.

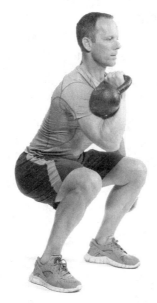

LEVEL 3

## ✴ Front squat

**BEST FOR:** any part of the program, any rep range. If you're an intermediate or advanced lifter, you may want to save the front squat for Hypertrophy and/or Strength & Power. But if you're planning to use the back squat for one of those programs, feel free to use the front squat anywhere else. Although it's impossible to quantify this, given the difference in limb lengths and thus form from one lifter to the next, Alwyn and many others believe it's the best exercise for developing your quadriceps. It allows a deeper range of motion than many of us can achieve with the back squat, and at the same time is widely considered safer for the knees. And because your torso is more upright than it would be on a back squat, it would seem that your posterior-chain muscles (especially the hamstrings) contribute less to the movement. This of course varies from lifter to lifter, and as noted in Chapter 2, studies haven't shown a difference in muscle activation between the back and front squat.

**GET READY**

- Set up a barbell in the squat rack just below shoulder height.
- Grab it with an overhand, shoulder-width grip, and rotate your arms under and around the bar until your upper arms are nearly parallel to the floor. The underside of your forearms will face the ceiling.
- Balance the bar on your front shoulders as you lift it off the supports. The bar will roll from your palms to your fingers as you balance it on your shoulders. As long as you keep your arms up and your torso upright, it'll stay in this spot.
- Step back from the rack and set your feet shoulder-width apart, with your toes pointed straight ahead or angled out slightly.

**MOVE**

- Push your hips back and lower your body until the tops of your thighs are parallel to the floor.
- Rise back up to the starting position.

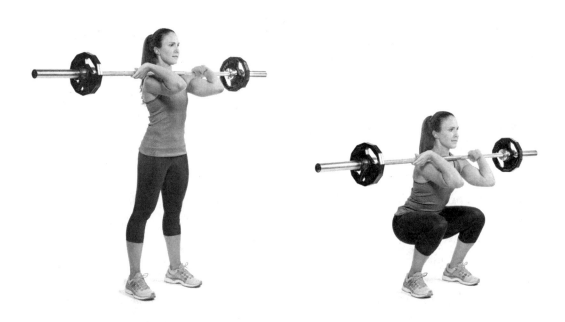

# ✳ Zercher squat

**BEST FOR:** an interesting, challenging novelty exercise for one of the programs in Basic Training or Hypertrophy, but not as a primary training exercise. It lowers your center of gravity, which puts you in position to lift a heavier load. But at the same time you're limited by the amount of weight your arms can support.

## GET READY

- First you have to decide which type of resistance you want to use. The barbell is easiest, which is why we show it here, but it's one Alwyn never uses with his clients; he prefers to use a sandbag, which isn't a strength challenge so much as a test of balance and grip endurance.

- Set the barbell up in a squat rack just below hip height. You need to either wrap the bar in a towel or pad, or start the exercise with a folded towel or piece of foam in the crook of your arms; otherwise, you're in for some seriously nasty abrasions.

- Squat down slightly and reach up to the bar with bent arms, resting the bar between your biceps and forearms. Lift the bar off the support and step back, holding it with your arms tight against your abdomen. Set your feet as you would for the front or goblet squat.

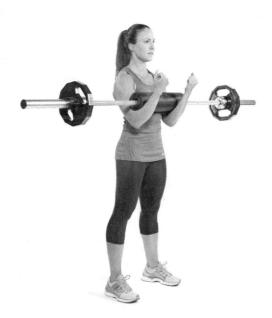

## MOVE

- Push your hips back, lowering your body as far as you can while keeping your torso as upright as possible.

- Rise back up to the starting position.

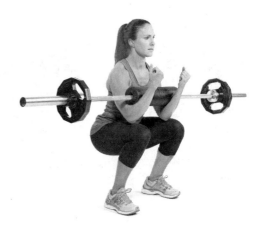

## LEVEL 3.5

## ✳ Offset overhead squat

**BEST FOR:** The combination of an overhead and off-center load makes this a fantastic core challenge, but not the best choice when the goal is to develop lower-body strength and size. I like to use it when the goal is fat loss or overall conditioning, but I confess I also use it when my knees are aching, no matter what my goal is. It gives you a way to work hard while putting hardly any compressive forces on your knee joints. Make sure you do the same number of reps with the weight on each side.

**GET READY**

- Grab a dumbbell or kettlebell and hold it overhead. If you're using a kettlebell (which we recommend), hold it against the outside of your forearm.
- Stand with your feet shoulder-width apart, with your toes pointed forward or angled out slightly.

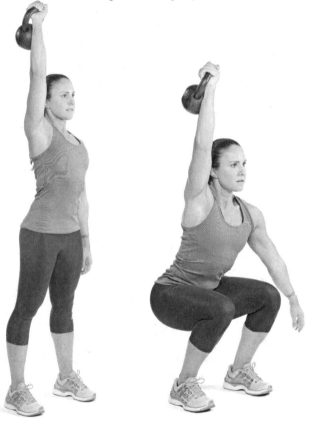

**MOVE**

- Push your hips straight back and descend until the tops of your thighs are parallel to the floor.
- Rise to the starting position.

## LEVEL 4

## ✳ Back squat

**BEST FOR:** strength, power, and muscle development. I say that with some hesitation, as it's a problematic exercise for some lifters, myself included. My back and knees just can't handle the compressive forces anymore. But, as probably the most-studied exercise for athletic training, it's linked directly with improved speed and jumping ability, and indirectly with higher-level achievement in strength and power sports like football. That is, the best players are typically stronger in the back squat than the less talented players. So if you can do the exercise with challenging weights and no joint pain during or after, it may offer the best path to develop lower-body strength and size.

### GET READY

- Set up a barbell in the squat rack just below shoulder height.
- Grab the bar overhand, your hands just outside shoulder width, and duck under the bar so it rests on your upper trapezius. If you squeeze your shoulder blades together, your upper traps will form a nice little shelf for the bar. (Technically, this is called an Olympic or high-bar squat, to distinguish it from the powerlifting version, where the bar is lower on your back, and your torso leans farther forward.)

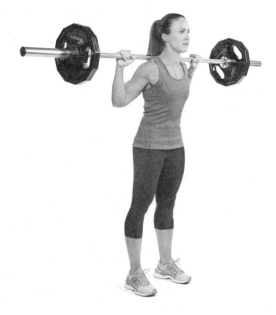

- Lift the bar off the supports and take a step back, setting your feet shoulder-width apart (you can also go a bit wider; the best position is whatever gives you the strongest platform and feels most natural), with your toes pointing forward or angled out slightly.

### MOVE

- Push your hips back and descend as far as you can without your heels coming off the floor or your lower back shifting out of its neutral position. Ideally, you want the tops of your thighs slightly below parallel to the floor.
- Return to the starting position.

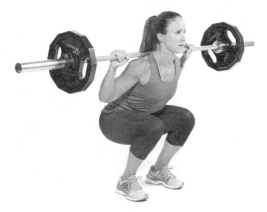

**SUPERCHARGE IT!**

## ✳ Hex-bar deadlift

**BEST FOR:** those who're strong but find the back squat problematic with the heavy loads required for the Strength & Power programs. Some of you just won't be good squatters no matter what. Perhaps your heels come off the floor, or you can't get your thighs parallel to the floor while keeping your lower back in the neutral position (a persistent problem for taller lifters—six-foot-two or above—who have longer limbs and thus more chances for something to go wrong). For many lifters, the hex-bar deadlift solves two big problems: It allows you to keep your heels on the floor, and thus keep the weight over the middle of your foot, aligned with your shoulders. Many of you will start a hex-bar deadlift with your thighs nearly parallel to the floor, which is as low as you'd get on a squat anyway. Thus, you're working the exact same muscles through the exact same range of motion, but probably with your back and torso in a safer, more upright position.

**GET READY**

- First, of course, you'll need a hex bar or a trap bar. (One is a six-sided hexagon, the other a four-sided trapezoid.) Remember that the weight of different bars can vary widely. The original trap bar, patented by Al Gerard, weighs 30 pounds. Some hex bars weigh 45 pounds, same as an Olympic barbell, but more heavy-duty bars, with high and low handles, could weigh more.
- If your gym has a bar with high and low handles, you have two choices: The low handles put the bar about 9 inches off the floor, which is the height of a conventional deadlift. The high handles are about 12 to 13 inches from the floor, which makes the exercise more like the rack deadlift shown in Chapter 9. It's probably better to use the low handles when using the hex-bar deadlift as a squat substitute, as that will set your hips and thighs lower at the start and finish and thus work them in a more squat-like way, with higher coactivation of your quadriceps and hamstrings.
- Stand in the middle of the bar with your feet shoulder-width apart and toes pointed straight ahead or angled out slightly.
- Reach down and grab the handles (your palms will be just outside your thighs and facing each other, in case that isn't obvious).
- Push your hips back, pull your shoulder blades down, and push your chest out. Tighten everything from hands to feet.

**MOVE**

- Thrust your hips forward as you pull the weight off the floor.
- Lower it under control to the floor. The heavier the weight, the less time you want to spend lowering it, which puts your back into a disadvantaged position. I put thin rubber mats on the floor so the plates don't make a loud noise when the bar lands.

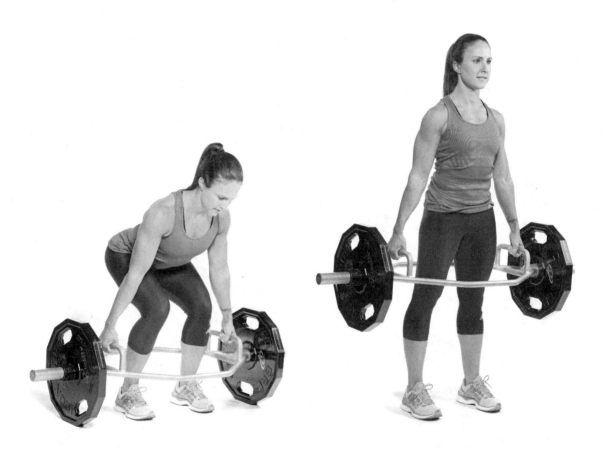

## LEVEL 5

✴ **Overhead squat**

**BEST FOR:**  I like to use this in fat-loss-oriented programs, especially Basic Training III or IV. It's a great movement for developing skill, mobility, and core and shoulder stability. Problem is, it's an advanced and technically complex exercise, so most readers won't be able to do it until later in the program, where it's not the best choice for either muscle or strength development. So for some readers it will work best the second time you do Basic Training. Advanced lifters, on the other hand, can drop it in wherever they choose.

**GET READY**

- Grab a barbell overhand with a very wide grip, probably double your shoulder width. Depending on your strength, you can start with the bar at shoulder height in a squat rack, which means you overhead press it to the starting position, or on

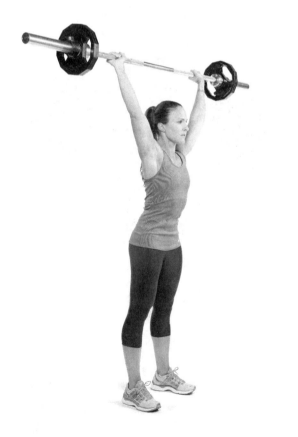
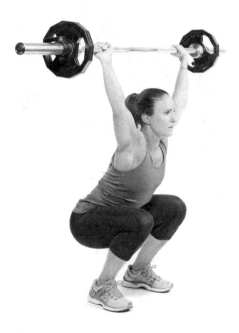

the floor, which means you pull it overhead however you're able. (You earn style points if you can do an Olympic snatch to get it overhead to begin.)

- Stand holding the barbell with straight arms over the back of your head. You're going to keep your arms straight and perpendicular to the floor throughout the movement. Set your feet shoulder-width apart; most of us will need to turn our toes out for this one.

**MOVE**

- Push your hips back and descend as far as you can while keeping your feet flat on the floor, your knees steady and aligned with your toes, and the bar over the back of your head, or slightly behind it.
- Push your hips forward as you return to the starting position.
- If you're new to the exercise, focus on improving your depth—going lower while maintaining perfect form and completing all the repetitions—before you worry about adding weight to the bar.

# Hinge

YOU NEVER FORGET YOUR FIRST ONE. The deadlift was the first exercise that made me feel like a real lifter. My knees were nearly shot by the time I started doing squats, and I was never very strong on the bench press. But with the deadlift I worked up to a max of twice my body weight, and although it scared the hell out of me (even with a thick weightlifting belt, it felt like important parts of me were coming apart), it gave me a sense of accomplishment.

In the years since, my concept of accomplishment has changed. Form and feel matter most to me now—doing each exercise right, and feeling it exactly where it should be felt. That's the key to success with the exercises in this chapter. I hope that everyone, even the most advanced lifters, will do the Level 1 exercise at least once in Basic Training I, and take your time moving up to Level 5. At each level, make sure you can feel the movement in your glutes and hamstrings, with minimal strain on your lower back. Just as important, make sure you feel the work equally on your left and right sides.

LEVEL 1

## ✴ Swiss-ball supine hip extension

**BEST FOR:** Basic Training I only. Everyone should try it at least once. If you can do 1 or 2 sets of 15 reps, great. You're ready for the higher-level exercises, and don't have to worry about this one again. If you can't do 15 reps, work on it until you can do 2 sets of 15 or until you finish Basic Training I, whichever comes first.

**GET READY**
- Lie on your back on the floor with your heels on a Swiss ball and your arms out to your sides.

**MOVE**
- Lift your hips until your body forms a straight line from your ankles to your neck.
- Lower your hips until they're close to but not touching the floor, and repeat until you finish the set.

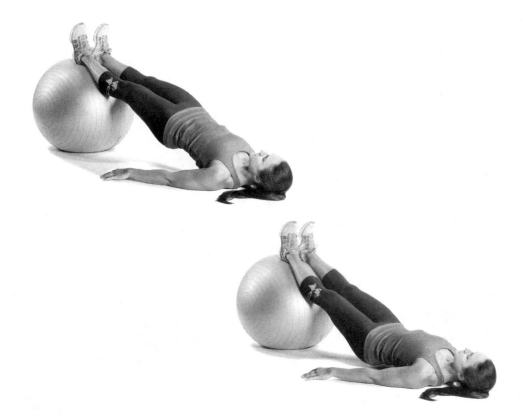

### LEVEL 1.5

## ✳ Supine hip extension with leg curl

**BEST FOR:** experienced lifters who try the supine hip extension and find it too easy for serious workouts. It's substantially more challenging for the simple reason that you're adding knee flexion to the movement. With hip extension—straightening your hips when they're bent forward—you generate force from the top of the muscle to the bottom. Bending or flexing your knee uses your hamstrings to generate force in the opposite direction, from bottom to top. A combination of the two movements makes each part harder than it would be on its own. As a bonus, you'll also work the gastrocnemius, the larger of the two main calf muscles, which helps bend the knee.

### GET READY

- You can use a Swiss ball, as shown on the bottom left and described; a suspension system like the TRX; or Valslides, as shown on the bottom right, which, according to my aching muscles, offers the toughest challenge.
- Lie on your back on the floor with your heels on the ball and your arms out to your sides.

### MOVE

- Lift your hips until your body forms a straight line from your ankles to your shoulders.
- At the same time, bend your knees and curl the ball toward your body until your feet are flat on the ball, your knees are bent about 90 degrees, and your body forms a straight line from knees to shoulders.
- Straighten your legs and lower your hips until they're close to but not touching the floor.

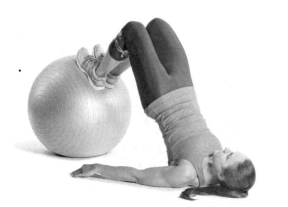
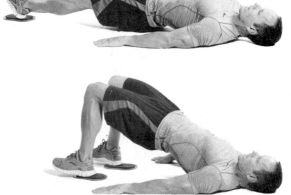

## LEVEL 2

✳ **Romanian deadlift**

**BEST FOR:** any program in Basic Training or Hypertrophy. It may be the best hinge exercise an experienced lifter can use for higher reps with a relatively heavy load. Some home-gym lifters will do this with dumbbells, and of course that's fine. But if you have a choice, I encourage you to use the barbell because your upper-back muscles—the trapezius and others that control your shoulder blades—will get fried. You'll notice those muscles working when you use a barbell for higher reps, but you'll *really* feel them when they're working to control two separate loads. Your traps may quit on you before you exhaust your glutes and hamstrings, which would limit the effectiveness of the exercise.

**GET READY**

- Set up a barbell in a rack so it's just above your knees.
- Grab the barbell with a shoulder-width, overhand grip, lift it off the rack, and step back, holding it with straight arms against the front of your thighs.
- Set your feet shoulder-width apart, toes pointed forward.

**MOVE**

- Push your hips back and lower the bar until it's below your knees. (More advanced lifters can lower it halfway down their shins.) Your knees will bend slightly.

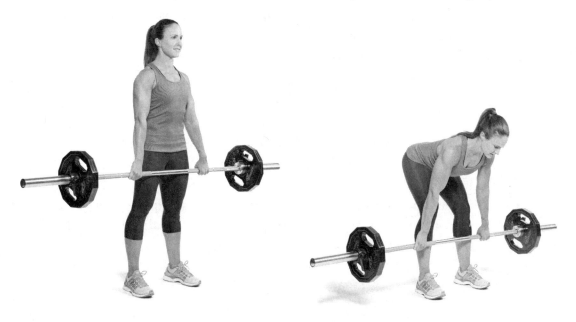

- Thrust your hips forward to raise the weight back to the starting position, keeping your arms straight and the bar close to (if not in contact with) your legs.

### LEVEL 2 ALTERNATIVE #1
## ✳ Cable pull-through

**BEST FOR:** higher-rep workouts in Basic Training. It's also good for home-gym lifters who use bands with a low attachment point (the bottom of a squat rack, for example). You'll find it offers a good way to load your glutes and hamstrings with minimal risk to the lower back . . . as long as you work with fairly light weights and control the tempo when you're lowering them. My own experience tells me it's not a good option with heavier weights and lower reps. The one time I tried it was one of the very few times I've left the gym with a sore back.

### GET READY

- Attach a rope handle to a low cable pulley. (It works the exact same way with a band attached to a pillar a few inches above the floor.)
- Stand with your back to the cable machine, feet just a bit beyond shoulder-width apart.
- Reach between your legs and grab the ends of the rope attachment. You may need to take a step forward so you start with tension on the cable.
- Set your body so your torso is bent forward at the hips (probably between a 45-degree angle to the floor and parallel to it), your back is flat, your knees are bent slightly, and your arms are straight. You want to feel like your glutes are "loaded," as if you're a swimmer in the Olympics and ready to dive off the platform to start the race.

### MOVE

- Thrust your hips forward as you straighten your body and pull the rope until your hands are just in front of your torso.
- Keep your back flat and arms straight throughout the movement.
- Remember that this isn't an exercise for your arms or shoulders. It's analogous to the kettlebell swing shown on page 219. It doesn't matter how far you pull the rope in front of your torso; you're only concerned with firing your hips and straightening your torso.

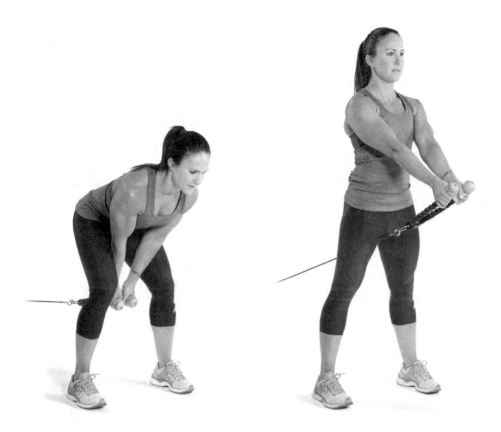

**LEVEL 2 ALTERNATIVE #2**

## ✳ Kettlebell or dumbbell sumo deadlift

**BEST FOR:** another high-rep alternative. It's especially useful if you're trying to minimize lower-back stress. It's not a great exercise for strength, power, and hypertrophy; you're putting your body in just about the strongest, safest position possible for generating maximum force, and then lifting a single weight that's a small fraction of what you could actually lift. That's why it never occurred to either of us to include it in an NROL book. But the further you go in Alwyn's *Supercharged* programs, the more you'll find yourself hard-pressed to find exercises you can do for high reps in a state of fatigue. For some readers this will be a viable exercise to use for Basic Training, assuming you have access to fairly heavy dumbbells or kettlebells. For others, it's something interesting to throw in for the highest-rep sets in Hypertrophy or even Strength & Power.

**GET READY**

- Set one or two kettlebells on the floor, or a heavy dumbbell resting upright.
- Stand over it with your feet spread wide apart and toes pointing out.
- It's hard to be precise about this, but the best position would probably put the center of the weight on a line with the balls of your feet.
- Bend over and grab the weight or weights with both hands. Use an overhand grip with the kettlebell(s), and with a dumbbell grab the upper end with your palms facing each other.
- Push your hips down and back slightly, pull your shoulders down, push your chest out, and tighten everything from hands to feet.

**MOVE**

- Thrust your hips forward to pull the weight(s) straight up from the floor.
- Lower the weight(s) to the floor and repeat.

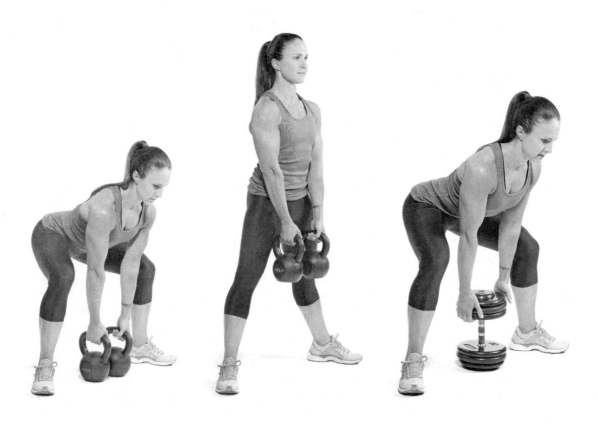

## LEVEL 3

# ✳ Rack deadlift

**BEST FOR:** lower-rep sets in Hypertrophy, and possibly even in Strength & Power. It's difficult, but not impossible, to do rack deadlifts for higher reps. The problem is that you need to set the bar down on the supports after each rep and reset your body. It's time-consuming, and your form will probably deteriorate anytime you go above 10 reps. You never want to do deadlifts without perfect form, whether you're lifting from a rack or the floor.

**GET READY**

- Set the pins or rails of a squat rack at or just below knee height.
- Set the Olympic barbell on the pins or rails and load it with weights. (If you don't have a rack, you can also lift from boxes, as long as you can find two boxes of equal height, and that height places the bar at or just below your knees.)
- Grab the bar overhand, with your hands just outside your knees.
- Push your hips back, pull your shoulder blades down, and push your chest out. Tighten everything from hands to feet.

**MOVE**

- Thrust your hips forward as you pull the weight off the supports and straighten your body.
- Lower it slowly to the pins or rails, reset your body, and repeat.

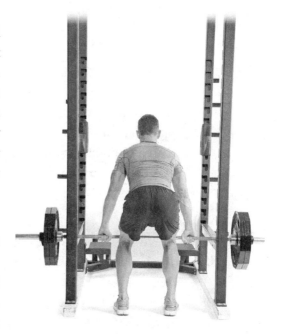

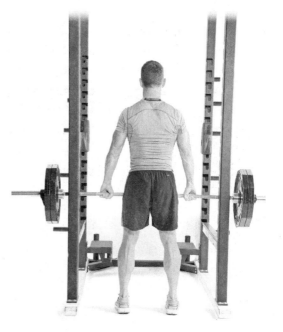

## LEVEL 4

## ✳ Deadlift

**BEST FOR:** max weights, low reps in Strength & Power I, II, and III. It can also work anywhere in Hypertrophy, although I wouldn't recommend it for the higher-rep sets. (For those, you can substitute another exercise that allows you to establish a rhythm, and doesn't require you to put the weight on the floor and reset your grip each time.) It's probably the best exercise we have for building and strengthening the posterior chain—glutes, hamstrings, spinal erectors (the parallel sets of muscles that run up your middle and lower back on either side of your spine), and trapezius—and is also great for improving your grip and the stability and strength of a long list of core muscles.

### GET READY

- Set a loaded bar on the floor and stand with your feet shoulder-width apart, toes pointed straight ahead or angled out slightly, and shins right up against the bar.
- Bend over and grab the bar overhand, with your hands just outside your legs.
- Push your hips back, pull your shoulders down, push your chest out, and tighten everything from hands to feet.

### MOVE

- Thrust your hips forward as you pull the weight off the floor, keeping it as close to your legs as possible.
- Lower it under control to the floor by pushing your hips back, and then bending at the knees after the bar passes them. You don't want to lose the natural arch in your lower back at any point when you're lifting or lowering the weight.
- Once the bar rests on the floor, relax, reset your grip, and reposition your body for the next rep. Don't do consecutive reps with heavy weights without getting your hips back, shoulders down, and chest up.

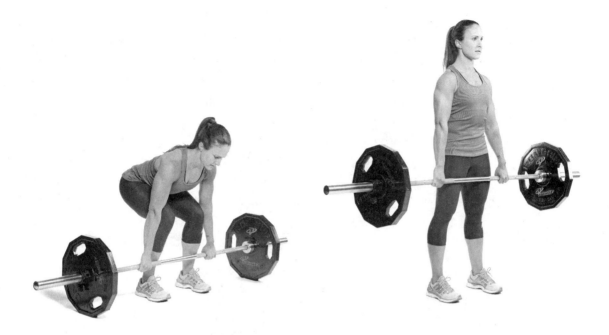

## Gripping Issues

At some point, your grip strength will become a limiting factor. I use chalk on my palms for almost every set of 10 reps or fewer, a practice most commercial gyms frown on, if they don't outlaw it altogether. (Planet Fitness doesn't allow deadlifts in the first place, so it's not an issue there.) If there's no posted rule against it at your gym, I recommend a cautious approach: First get a brick of gym chalk—you can buy a pound of magnesium carbonite at performbetter.com for $15—and then break off a sliver. Put that in a soap container with a lid. Rub it on your palms right before each set. When you're finished, wipe off your hands as well as the bar. If you drop a crumb or two on the floor, wipe those up as well. That way, even if it's against the rules, a gym employee who sees you using chalk may cut you a break for being both subtle and considerate.

## SUPERCHARGE IT!

For the heaviest sets in Strength & Power II and III (and possibly S&P I as well), you'll want to use the mixed grip. That is, one hand under the bar, one hand over. Usually the dominant hand—your right if you're right-handed—goes over the bar while the nondominant hand goes under. Women and some men with small hands may prefer to use this on most deadlift sets.

One caution: With the mixed grip, it's more important than ever to keep the bar as close to your body as possible throughout the lift, even if it means scraping your shins from time to time. If the bar gets out in front, the mixed grip could cause some twisting, which is the last thing you want with a heavy weight.

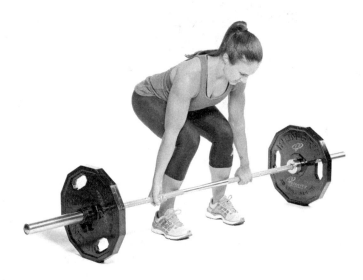

### LEVEL 4 ALTERNATIVE #1

## ✳ Sumo deadlift

**BEST FOR:** The conventional deadlift favors those with long arms relative to their legs and torso. Those with relatively long legs or torso might have trouble getting into, and staying in, a strong, safe position for the lift. A sumo deadlift allows the long-legged lifter to shorten his or her legs by spreading them out wide. A lifter with a long torso gets to start in a more upright posture, potentially reducing the risk of back strain. You should see more development of your quadriceps and hip adductors—the inner-thigh muscles with cool names like *magnus* and *longus* (and slightly wimpier ones like *brevis* and *minimus*).

**GET READY**

- Set a loaded bar on the floor and stand with your feet as wide as possible, toes pointed out, and shins right up against the bar.
- Bend over and grab the bar overhand (or with a mixed grip, on your heaviest sets), with your arms just inside your legs and hands about shoulder-width apart.
- Push your hips down and back slightly, pull your shoulders down, push your chest out, and tighten everything from hands to feet.

**MOVE**

- Thrust your hips forward as you pull the weight off the floor, keeping it as close to your legs as possible.
- Lower it under control to the floor.

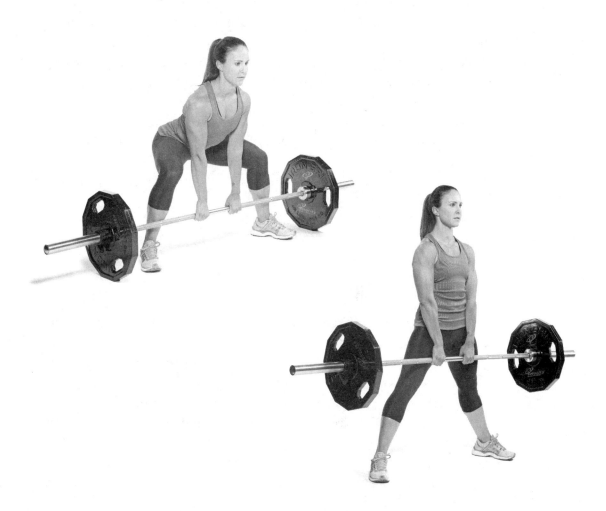

## ✳ Hex-bar deadlift

In the previous chapter I included the hex-bar deadlift with the squats, which is how Alwyn uses it with his clients. However, some of you will want to use it here, with the deadlifts, and there's absolutely no problem with that.

A 2011 study in the *Journal of Strength and Conditioning Research* compared the hex-bar deadlift to the conventional deadlift with a straight bar, using nineteen experienced male powerlifters (average weight: 252 pounds) to test the exercises. Their average one-rep max was 538 pounds in the conventional deadlift and 583 pounds with a hex bar—an 8 percent difference. The extra strength with the hex bar comes from two different directions: There's less stress on the lower back, which minimizes a lifter's weakest link, and there's more involvement of the quadriceps, which help the hamstrings and glutes.

Open question: If you use the hex bar, and it allows you to use heavier weights than you could with a conventional or sumo deadlift, does that automatically translate to increased size and strength? I don't think we can say, and I'm not sure it matters a lot. Heavy squats and deadlifts, with any style, should give you the best chance to achieve whatever muscle and performance level your genetics and training intensity allow.

As someone with bad knees but a strong back, I've always preferred the conventional style. But there's really no wrong choice. Try them all and use the one that gives you the best performance with the least discomfort.

### LEVEL 5

## ✳ Wide-grip deadlift

**BEST FOR:** any of the Hypertrophy programs, with high or low reps. Advanced lifters can also use it when doing Basic Training with a fat-loss emphasis. I find it works best when you do fast reps, stopping just short of tapping the weights on the floor. But it can also work just fine as a traditional deadlift, using heavy weights and stopping to reset your grip and posture on each rep. However you use it, it both requires and develops all of these fitness qualities: ankle and hip mobility; core strength and stability; strength, endurance, and stability in your scapular stabilizers (the trapezius, rhomboids, and other muscles responsible for moving your shoulder blades, or holding them in place when you need them to *not* move); grip strength and endurance. That's on top of the strength and endurance you need in your hamstrings, glutes, and spinal erectors, and to a lesser extent in your quadriceps (the knee angle is more severe than in a conventional deadlift, which means your quads will contribute more to the lift).

**GET READY**

- Set a loaded bar on the floor and stand with your feet shoulder-width apart, toes pointed straight ahead or angled out slightly, and shins right up against the bar.
- Bend over and grab the bar overhand, with your hands about twice shoulder-width apart.
- Push your hips back, pull your shoulders down, push your chest out, and tighten everything from hands to feet.

**MOVE**

- Thrust your hips forward as you pull the weight off the floor, keeping it as close to your legs as possible.
- Lower it under control to the floor by pushing your hips back, and then bending at the knees after the bar passes them.
- If you're doing 10 or more reps, stop just short of the floor, and go right into the next lift. If you're doing fewer than 10, set the bar down and reset your grip and starting position.

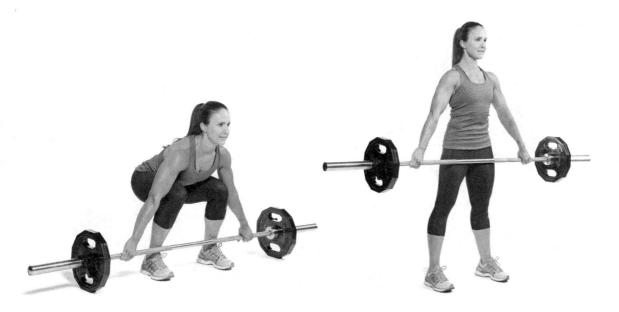

SUPERCHARGE IT!

## ✳ Wide-grip deadlift from deficit

**BEST FOR:** advanced lifters with exceptional hip mobility, back strength, and core stability who want an extremely challenging exercise for one or two programs in Basic Training or Hypertrophy.

### GET READY/MOVE

- You have two choices for creating a deficit:
  - You can stand on one or two weight plates, putting your feet an inch or two above the floor. You would start each repetition from a dead stop, with the weight on the floor, just like a conventional deadlift.
  - You can stand on a low box, and do continuous repetitions without setting the weight on the floor. In this version, which is more of a Romanian deadlift with an extreme range of motion than a traditional deadlift, you want to pick the weight up off the floor, step up to the box, and then on each repetition lower the weight until the edges of the weight plates are an inch or two below the level of the box.

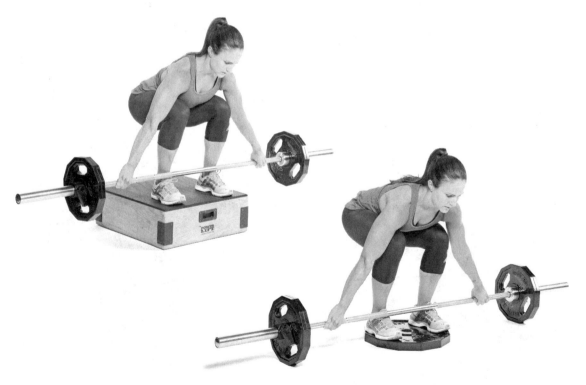

# Push

THE PUSH-UP IS THE FIRST TRAINING exercise most of us learn, or at least the first movement pattern that isn't based on something we do for fun, like running, jumping, climbing, or swimming. You understand from the get-go that it's a test of your strength and overall fitness. Interestingly, when I coached kids, they couldn't wait to show me how many push-ups they could do. They didn't object to getting down on the grass or floor and pushing themselves not just beyond their comfort zone, but beyond their previous performance. To them, *it's the entire point.* One time, when I was coaching a team of eleven- and twelve-year-old girls, two of my players got into an impromptu push-up contest. (It wasn't part of my practice plan for preteen soccer players.) They refused to quit until one had beaten the other. Their form was pretty atrocious, as you can imagine, but once both of them went beyond 30 reps, it didn't matter.

I think both girls learned an important lesson that day: You never know what you can do until you try it. Now I wish I could find a way to get that lesson across to all the people in health clubs who'll use a seated chest-press machine workout after workout, year after year, without once getting down on the floor and doing a push-up.

If two of my *Twilight*-reading soccer players could do more than 30, don't you think you can do at least one?

My disdain for chest-press machines, while pure and radiant, is nothing compared to my absolute hatred of shoulder-press machines. I get why chest-press machines exist. People equate push-ups with punishment and pain, and the best-known free-weight version of the exercise, the bench press, looks like a suicide pact, with that loaded barbell poised over your trachea like a guillotine. (As some of you know, there's a version of the exercise called the guillotine press, in which you deliberately lower the bar to your throat. Be grateful that Alwyn would rather drop a weight on his own foot than include it in his programs.) But why in the world would someone even bother to invent a shoulder-press machine? What's so hard about lifting a couple of dumbbells over your shoulders?

Another story: A few months after the push-up contest, my wife asked me to do a presentation on exercise and fitness for our daughter's Girl Scout troop. Again, the girls were all eleven or twelve, but unlike the athletes on my soccer team, this group had a huge range of shapes, sizes, and fitness levels. I brought along a pair of 10-pound dumbbells to demonstrate some exercises. As soon as I set them down, the girls ran to the weights and tried to lift them overhead, even though I never suggested it, and didn't really think most of them could do it.

Out of perhaps a dozen girls, how many do you think were able to lift those 10-pound dumbbells overhead?

If you guessed "all of them," you're right (and you've probably heard me tell this story before). It wasn't just the big girl playing soccer and basketball on elite travel teams. It wasn't just my daughter, the "loser" of the push-up contest at soccer practice. (She collapsed after 32 or 33, while the other girl got one more.) It wasn't just the girls who were more physically mature. All of them did it, and most did it for multiple reps.

As frustrated as I get when I look around the gym and see healthy men and women wasting time on machines that replicate the push-up and shoulder press when they would get far more benefit from doing the actual exercises, I know that machines are here to stay. What I don't get is why so many people in the weight room, the ones who understand that it's smarter to work with dumbbells, don't bother challenging themselves. It's mind-boggling to see adults press weights that I know from firsthand experience would barely challenge a Girl Scout.

But all of them—the machinists as well as the timid free-weighters—would be better served by focusing on the push-up, an exercise many haven't even attempted since childhood. You'll find lots of options on the following pages, starting with the classic version. Alwyn could write an entire book on push-ups and still not exhaust all the variations he knows. The one thing we can't include: two vampire-loving pre-teen girls to make you feel foolish for avoiding this exercise. Really, it's child's play.

## LEVEL 1
### ✳ Push-up

**BEST FOR:** everybody should do push-ups in Basic Training I. More experienced lifters can do a horizontal variation in one workout and a vertical push-up in the other. Those with less experience can use basic push-ups in both workouts. The only exception to the push-up rule for Basic Training I is for a male lifter who can do 2 sets of at leasts 15 reps of any push-up variation in this chapter. That includes everything in Levels 1 and 3. Of course, by the time you figure out if you can do all of them, you'll probably be finished with Basic Training I anyway. (Devious, I know.) For female lifters the same rule applies, although for personal reasons I'd rather you didn't move on just yet. The gym would be a better place if more women were seen cranking out push-ups, especially the advanced versions.

**GET READY**

- Get into push-up position: arms straight down from your shoulders and perpendicular to the floor, feet close together, weight resting on your hands and toes, and your body straight from neck to ankles.

**MOVE**

- Lower your chest until it's within an inch of the floor or your upper arms are even with your shoulder blades, whichever happens first.
- Push back up to the starting position.

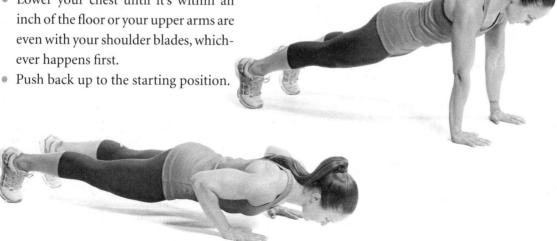

### Modify It

If you can't do at least 10 traditional push-ups, use the push-up with hands elevated in Basic Training I. Set your hands on a surface that's high enough to allow you to hit double-digit repetitions, but not so high that the exercise is easy. For most women and some men, a bench or box that's 12 to 18 inches off the floor will do the trick. It's also a good use for the Smith machine, if your gym has one. Set the barbell at the lowest level that allows you to get all the prescribed reps. Your goal is to lower the bar over time, and eventually get down to the floor for your push-ups.

### But Don't . . .

Do the "girl" push-up, with your knees on the floor. It minimizes the two biggest benefits to the traditional push-up, as opposed to chest presses with a machine or free weights:

1. It allows your shoulder blades to operate without the restriction they'd have if you were lying on your back doing a bench press.
2. Your core muscles come into play to stabilize your spine and pelvis.

When you're on your knees you're probably going to shrug your shoulders up, which restricts your shoulder blades. (This will also happen when you do the push-up with hands elevated, but to a lesser extent; that's why it's important to use the lowest possible angle.) And your core muscles have hardly any challenge. Even worse, it offers no direct path to performing the traditional exercise. Nobody goes from push-ups on the knees to the classic push-up on the toes, but everybody who works at the push-up with hands elevated should eventually work their way down to the floor.

### SUPERCHARGE IT!

If you can do 2 sets of at least 15 traditional push-ups, follow this progression to find the variation that will push you to your limit:

1. Stack your feet, resting one on top of the other; switch feet each set.
2. Elevate your feet on a step or bench.
3. Raise one leg; do equal reps with one leg elevated.
4. Elevate one foot on a step or bench, and raise the other next to it but without support; do equal reps with each foot on the step.

5. Put your feet on an unstable object, like a Swiss ball.

6. Elevate your feet with a suspension system.

7. Elevate one foot on a Swiss ball, and hold the other one up alongside it but without support; do equal reps with each foot on the ball.

8. Elevate one foot with a suspension system, and raise the other next to it; do equal reps with each foot suspended (this is a current favorite, and a real ass-kicking core exercise).

9. Put your hands on an unstable surface, like a foam pad or Bosu ball.

10. Put one hand on a medicine ball and the other on the floor (do equal reps with each hand on the ball).

11. Put both hands on a medicine ball (shown below).

12. Put each hand on a medicine ball of the same size.

13. Lower your chest and shoulders toward one hand, then the other; each push-up counts as a repetition.

14. Lift your right knee toward your right elbow, then your left knee toward your left elbow (Spiderman push-up); each push-up counts as a repetition.

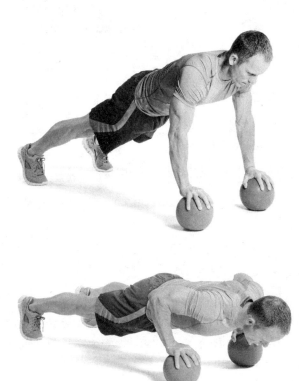

**Vertical Options**

You can try these push-up variations in any program in Basic Training or Hypertrophy when you're looking for a vertical option.

## ✳ Jackknife push-up

Start in the push-up position, but lift your hips as high as you can, forming a V shape with your torso. Your heels will be off the floor. Lower yourself as far as you can without banging your head on the floor, then push back up.

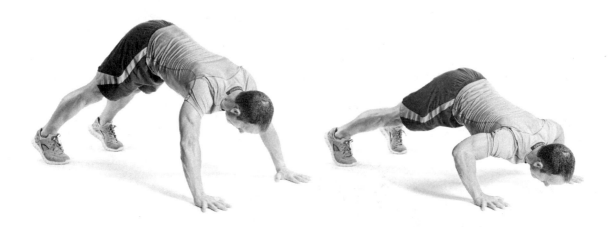

## ✳ Jackknife push-up with elevated feet

Same exercise, only with your toes resting on a box or bench that's 18 to 24 inches high.

## ✳ Modified handstand push-up

Two choices: With your back to a wall, bend over and set your hands on the floor. Walk your feet up the wall, and scoot your hands in as close to the wall as possible. Do as many push-ups as you can, getting your head as close to the floor as you dare. The other option is to stack boxes as high as you can, resting your toes on the top one.

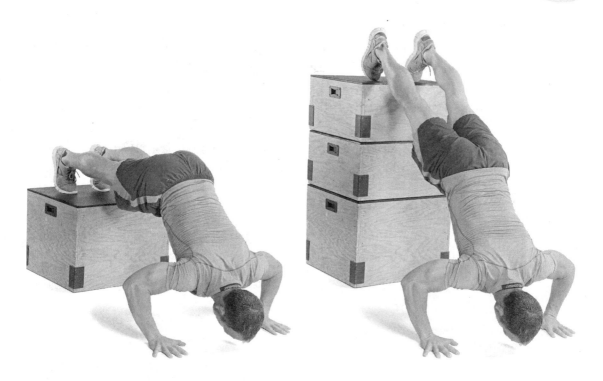

## LEVEL 2

✳ **Standing single-arm cable chest press**

**BEST FOR:** I think this is an amazing exercise for intermediate to advanced lifters to use for high reps in Basic Training II, III, or IV. Less experienced lifters can use it for Basic Training or Hypertrophy. Since you're using one arm at a time, your core works hard to prevent rotation. And, speaking as someone whose shoulders don't allow me to do some of the most popular pushing exercises, I love the fact that cable chest presses never hurt. The only drawback is loading: Eventually, stronger lifters won't be able to stay upright and balanced with weights that are heavy enough to provide a training stimulus.

**GET READY**

- Attach a stirrup handle to the cable apparatus, and move the pulley down to about chest level. (You can also use a band or tubing.)
- Grab the handle with your right hand and your back to the machine, and step out so there's tension on the cable when you hold the handle next to your shoulder.
- Stand with your left foot forward and right foot back, shoulders square and facing forward, and your torso braced and leaning forward slightly from the hips.

**MOVE**

- Push the handle straight out from your shoulder, keeping your shoulders square as you resist rotation.
- Do all your reps with your right arm, then switch arms and legs (right leg forward when you work your left side) and repeat the set.

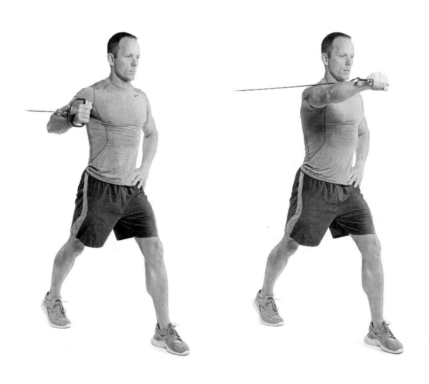

# ✳ Half-kneeling single-arm cable chest press

**BEST FOR:** I don't know how big a progression this is from the standing press, if it's a progression at all. But I think it allows advanced lifters to work with somewhat heavier weights before gravity tells you it's time to move on.

## GET READY

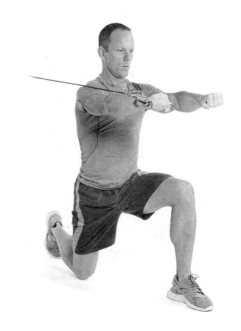

- Attach a stirrup handle to the cable apparatus, and move the pulley down to about hip level. (You can also use a band or tubing.)
- Grab the handle with your right hand and your back to the machine, and step out so there's tension on the cable when you hold the handle next to your shoulder.
- Kneel with your left foot forward and your right knee on the floor. (You may want to put a pad under your knee.)
- Unlike the standing version, you want to start with both arms extended out in front of you and aligned with each other as well as the cable or band. Your shoulders are still square and facing forward, and your torso is braced.
- Also unlike the standing press, you want to start with your torso upright, and keep it that way throughout the movement.

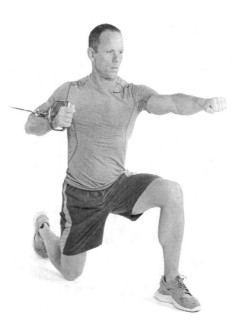

## MOVE

- Bring the handle back to your shoulder, keeping your nonworking arm straight out in front of you.
- Push the handle back to the starting position.
- Do all your reps with your right arm, then switch arms and legs (kneeling on your left knee when you work your left side) and repeat the set.

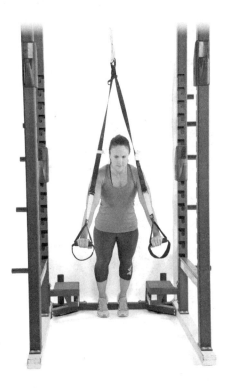

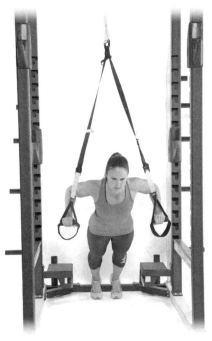

## LEVEL 2.5

# ✳ Push-up with hands suspended

**BEST FOR:** a metabolic boost combined with serious core training. The execution is so difficult, I'm not sure if someone strong and stable enough to do the exercise for double-digit reps will build much muscle or strength. But it's difficult in a good way, meaning it requires more effort than just about any pushing exercise I know (except for the one I describe next). So it's great for experienced lifters to use for fat loss in Basic Training.

### GET READY

- Set up a suspension system so the handles are 12 to 24 inches above the floor. Higher is easier; lower is harder.
- Grab the handles and get into push-up position, with your toes on the floor and your body mostly straight. (Even advanced lifters tend to hike their hips up a bit.)

### MOVE

- Lower yourself until your upper arms are parallel to the floor, then push back to the starting position.
- When you can do all the required reps, make it harder by lowering the handles.

## Especially Frustrating Alternative

The push-up with your hands on a Swiss ball is one of the hardest variations I've ever tried. I never get better at it, and it tends to hurt my shoulders, something that rarely happens with push-ups. But it's certainly an option if you like a challenge.

## LEVEL 3

✳ **T push-up**

**BEST FOR:** This is another one Alwyn has now used in all five books. It offers a metabolic boost for more advanced readers in Basic Training, and a very good challenge for everyone else in either Basic Training or Hypertrophy. The *Supercharged* version of the exercise, using dumbbells, means you can raise or lower the intensity for high or low reps.

**GET READY**

- Get into push-up position.

**MOVE**

- Lower your chest toward the floor, and as you push back up, twist to your right so your right arm comes off the floor and finishes straight over your left arm. In this position your body will form a T.
- Twist back and immediately begin your next push-up.
- As you push back up, twist to the left, so your left arm ends up over your right.
- Remember that each T push-up counts as a repetition. So if the workout calls for 15 per set, you'll have to do either 14 or 16 to get the same number to each side. If you stop at an odd number, no problem; just start the next set to the opposite side.

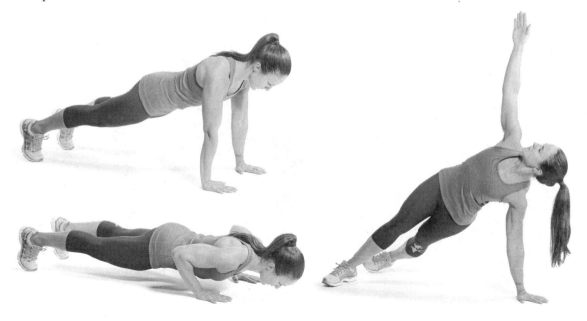

## SUPERCHARGE IT!

To do the T push-up with weights, you have two options:

1. Use a single dumbbell, of any type, and hold it in your working hand. Do the push-up the usual way, and lift the weight overhead at the top. Do half your reps, then switch sides and do the rest with the other hand.
2. Use two hexagonal dumbbells, and alternate sides for each repetition.

## LEVEL 4

## ✳ Dumbbell bench press

**BEST FOR:** pure muscle and strength. I hope most readers will use the push-up variations and cable chest press for Basic Training I through IV, and that less experienced readers will continue using them through most of Hypertrophy. But for experienced lifters, this is the go-to exercise for Hypertrophy, and it's the exercise Alwyn and I recommend for everyone who moves on to Strength & Power.

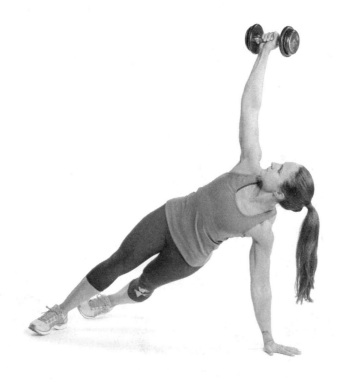

**GET READY**

- Grab a pair of relatively heavy dumbbells and lie on your back on a flat or incline bench. (My ego prefers the flat bench, but my shoulders think my ego is a bad influence, and force me to use the incline.)
- Hold the weights straight up over your shoulders, with your feet planted flat on the floor, shoulder-width apart. If your feet don't reach the floor when the bench is flat, either incline the bench, or better yet, skip this exercise altogether. The bench press, like the push-up, is a total-body exercise. You need feet on the floor to give you a solid foundation for lifting heavy weights. If you're going to put your feet on the bench, you're only slightly better off than you would be on a chest-press machine.

**MOVE**

- Lower the weights toward the edges of your shoulders. Those with long arms may want to stop when your upper arms are even with your shoulder blades; it's probably better for your long-term shoulder health.
- Press the weights straight up toward the ceiling.

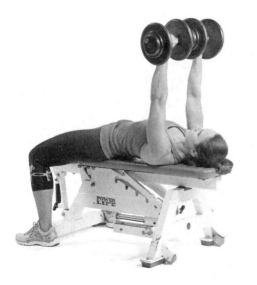
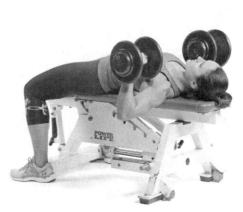

## LEVEL 4.1

# ✳ Dumbbell single-arm bench press

**BEST FOR:** one of the Hypertrophy programs, or for any program in Basic Training your second time through. It's a terrific exercise, and with practice you probably won't have to use significantly less weight than you lift on the bilateral version for the same number of reps. As with any unilateral movement, you're doing double the number of reps designated by the template, which makes it a good metabolic stimulus as well as a solid core-training exercise.

### GET READY

- Grab a dumbbell and lie on your back on a flat or incline bench. If you just finished a program using a flat bench, I recommend shifting to the incline.
- Hold the weight straight up over your chest, with your feet planted flat on the floor, shoulder-width apart, and your nonworking hand on your stomach.
- Traditionally, I recommend starting with your nondominant side—your left if you're right-handed. Recently, though, a couple of trainers have suggested starting with the dominant arm. When you start with your weaker arm, your stronger arm never gets fully challenged. But if you start with the stronger arm, and do a challenging set to the point of fatigue, then your weaker side has to work a lot harder to complete the same number of reps. I find it's much more exhausting to train this way, which means it probably accomplishes more.

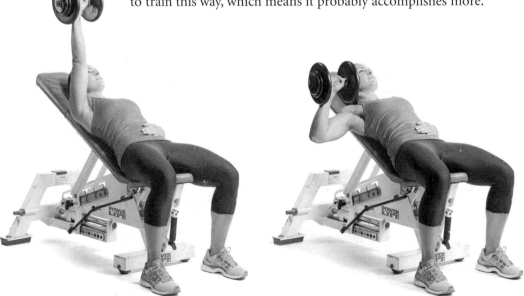

**MOVE**

- Lower the weight toward the edge of your shoulder, and press back to the starting position.
- Do all your reps and repeat with the other arm.

## LEVEL 5

## ✳ Dumbbell shoulder press

**BEST FOR:** developing pure muscle and strength on a vertical plane. You may think it's odd to put the "advanced" label on an exercise that, as I wrote in the introduction to this chapter, any twelve-year-old thinks is the first thing you should do with a dumbbell. Alwyn sees a sharp distinction between what you "can" and "should" do. Trainers will typically have beginners do the shoulder press while seated on a bench or, worse, sitting with their backs braced against a vertical support. In Alwyn's view, anybody who does the exercise should be able to do it standing up. Like the push-up and bench press, it's a total-body exercise. Novice lifters won't have the core or shoulder stability and strength to do it with good form.

**GET READY**

- Grab a pair of dumbbells and stand holding them in front of your shoulders, with your feet shoulder-width apart. You can turn your palms in if that's easier on your shoulders, or hold them the conventional way, with your palms forward.

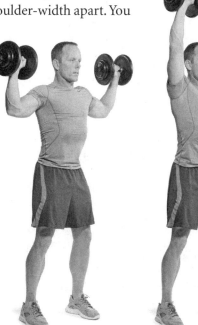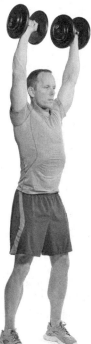

**MOVE**

- Press the weights straight up.
- Lower them to the starting position and repeat.

### SUPERCHARGE IT!

The single-arm shoulder press is a good challenge to your core stability, and offers a nice little metabolic stimulus. It should work best for stronger lifters using relatively heavy weights. Even trickier: hold two dumbbells, and alternate arms.

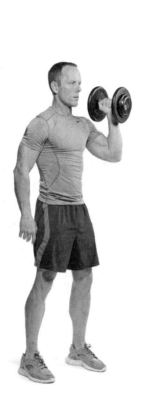 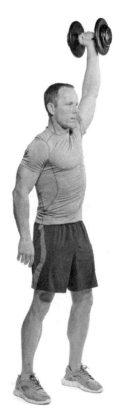

### LEVEL 7.5

## ✳ Barbell bench press

**BEST FOR:** competitive lifters. As Alwyn told me when we were writing this chapter, "Other than ego, I'm not sure it actually does much for the general-population trainee. You can get more metabolic work with other exercises, and can work your core and other muscles with push-up variations. There's more range of motion with dumbbell work, so that's a better hypertrophy choice. All those options are less stressful on the shoulders. The flat barbell bench press pretty much wrecks every shoulder joint eventually." The key word there is "eventually." You lessen the risk by using the exercise as part of your training program, rather than the focus of it. Even Alwyn uses it for a few weeks here and there in his own training. I assume that every experienced lifter reading this has done it, many still do, and many who haven't before will want to by the time they reach Strength & Power. All I ask is that you be careful, give yourself long breaks from the exercise, and back off when your shoulders feel worse from one workout to the next.

## GET READY

- Load a barbell and lie on your back on a flat or incline bench with your feet shoulder-width apart and flat on the floor. Grab the bar overhand with your hands about one and a half times shoulder-width apart.
- Lift the bar off the supports, or have a spotter lift it off for you on low-rep sets, and hold it straight over your chest.
- Tighten up everything, from your feet to your hands. You want your feet directly beneath your knees and angled out slightly. Your lower back is arched, your core is tight, and your shoulder blades are pulled together in back. Grab the bar like an iron dishrag you're trying to wring out.

## MOVE

- Lower the bar to your lower chest, keeping your upper arms close to your torso. Don't let your elbows flare out; you'll put more strain on your shoulders.
- Push the bar back up to the starting position, keeping your shoulder blades pulled together in back. You should feel your entire body pushing the weight, including your legs, as if you were standing up and pushing a car out of ditch.

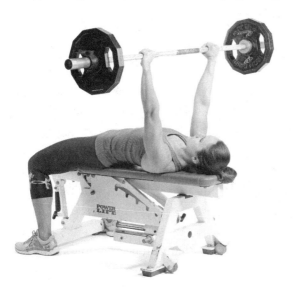
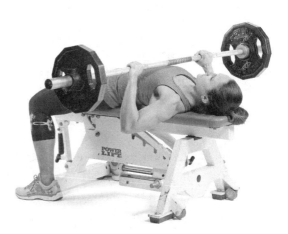

## Acceptable Variations

You can use a closer grip, with your thumbs perhaps 12 to 15 inches apart, for more triceps work. You can also do a board press, with one or two pieces of 2-by-4 set flat on your sternum. If you use two, you can tape them together. (A thick phone book works just as well.) The idea is to shorten the range of motion, emphasizing lockout strength, which is more dependent on your triceps. It's probably easier on your shoulders as well.

## Other Variations

Powerlifters and other strength athletes use bands and chains as part of their training on the bench press, squat, and deadlift. I assume they help, since the powerlifters I know are extremely analytical; if they didn't see a direct cause and effect with those training tools, I doubt if they'd use them for long. Alwyn doesn't use them, even when training powerlifters, so we don't include them here.

## Other Push Exercises

We've left out several popular pushing exercises:

## ✳ Dip

Because your upper arms are behind your torso while pushing your body weight, it's a brutal exercise for your shoulder joints.

## ✳ Dumbbell fly

Bodybuilders love this exercise, in which you hold two dumbbells over your chest, lower them out to your sides, and then pull them back. I once found myself in an argument with a bodybuilder who was convinced the exercise does something you can't get from a mix of bench presses and push-ups. I argued that the action at the shoulder joints isn't appreciably different. You're just changing the angle of your elbows so the weights are farther away from your torso at the bottom. The tradeoff is that you have to use lighter weights, and even then you're putting more strain on your shoulders. At least one study confirms that it activates the same muscles in the same way, and also shows that it activates them for less time than barbell or dumbbell bench presses, making it an inferior exercise.

## ✳ Floor press

You lie on the floor and do barbell or dumbbell chest presses, with the floor stopping your descent and thus shortening the range of motion. This one is more popular with powerlifters than regular gym rats, and again, I'll take their word that it helps improve their competitive lifts. If anything, it hurts my shoulders more than traditional bench presses.

## ✳ Decline bench press

Bodybuilders use this one interchangeably with dips, with the idea that it better activates the lower fibers of the pectoralis major. We know that incline bench presses give more work to the upper part of the pec major (the clavicular portion), while the middle part (sternocostal) gets more action on the flat bench. The open question is whether it's worth the effort to target those lower fibers, which originate at the top of the external obliques. Bodybuilders are convinced you need specialized exercises to develop the lower pecs, but for the rest of us, it's hard to justify taking extra time for so little muscle.

# 11

# Pull

IN MY PREVIOUS LIFE as a magazine fitness editor I encountered an odd problem from time to time: a model who looked great from the front or sides—magnificent abs, chest, shoulders, arms—but looked ordinary from the back. A fit guy, to be sure, but not particularly strong or well trained. It was easy to understand why. Nobody pays a fitness model for his trapezius.

The guys who do get paid for their traps—the diamond-shaped upper-back muscle that's responsible for moving your shoulder blades up, down, and in—are the no-neck bodybuilders, who do shoulder shrugs with weights the size of compact cars to build mounds of contractile tissue where the rest of us have open space.

That's why it's such a challenge to convince guys to invest as much time on pulling exercises as they spend on their chest, abs, and biceps. It's a somewhat easier sell for women, who seem to have a more acute appreciation of line of sight. They understand that people look at you from every angle, not just the ones you can see in your own mirror.

For either gender, pulling exercises offer your best hope to counteract the dual forces of technology and gravity. Spend too much time hunched over various iThings and your posture will suffer. You'll look tired and defeated even if you're at the top of your game.

I noted in Chapter 7 that Alwyn includes a pull in every workout. You'll typically choose a rowing exercise (a horizontal pull) in your A workout and a pulldown or chin-up (vertical pull) in the B workout. Both types of pulls work the same back muscles—primarily the latissimus dorsi (lats) and trapezius, along with the rear shoulders and biceps. But they use them in slightly different ways. With a horizontal pull, your trapezius retracts your shoulder blades, pulling them together toward your spine. The middle part of the trapezius does most of the work. On a vertical pull, the lower part of the trapezius acts to pull and rotate the shoulder blades down and in.

And what about the shoulder shrug, the exercise that turns the upper trapezius into the muscular speed bumps favored by bodybuilders? Alwyn, like most strength coaches these days, thinks it's best left to those whose living depends on having massive upper traps. There's really no reason for anyone else to waste time on heavy shrugs. Your goal, in fact, is to keep your shoulder blades *down* on pulling exercises. (The exception is on Olympic lifts, which we'll discuss in Chapter 16.) This is especially tricky for the youngest and oldest novice lifters, whose shoulders tend to rise because they don't yet have the strength and coordination to control them. On any pull, including the deadlifts shown in Chapter 9, your strongest and safest position is one in which you keep your shoulder blades down and pull them together at the end of the lift.

## LEVEL 1
## ✳ Standing cable row

**BEST FOR:** It's the best horizontal pull for novice lifters, for two big reasons. Since you're on your feet, you engage just about every muscle you have to keep you upright and prevent your torso from rotating. And because of the constant tension provided by the cable or band, you get a feel for the muscles working in your upper back, rear shoulders, biceps, and forearms that you may not get with free-weight exercises. I encourage even the most advanced lifters to start with this one in Basic Training I, when you're doing sets of 15 reps. The exercise becomes more problematic when you work with heavier weights and lower reps; even when you're strong enough to handle the load, you won't be able to brace yourself in the standing position.

**GET READY**

- Set the pulley of a cable machine to waist height, and attach a stirrup handle.
- Grab the handle in your nondominant hand and step back so you're facing the machine with your arm fully extended in front of you.
- Set your feet shoulder-width apart, with your toes pointed forward, knees and hips bent slightly, chest up, and shoulders square—that is, aligned with your feet. Rest your nonworking hand behind your back or on your thigh or hip.
- Tighten your hip and torso muscles to brace your core.

**MOVE**

- Pull the handle to the side of your torso, keeping your shoulders square and minimizing upper-body rotation.
- Return to the starting position, do all your reps, switch arms, and repeat the set with your other arm.

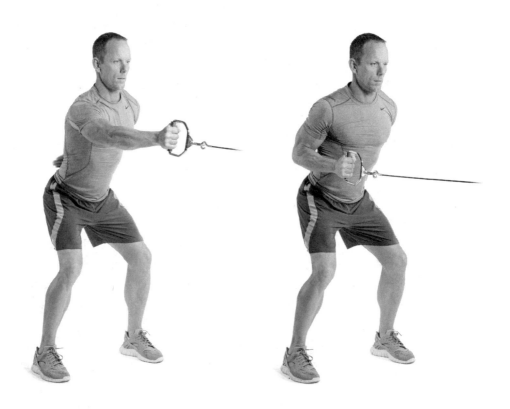

## SUPERCHARGE IT!

Alwyn uses four variations on the basic standing row. Remember that you're doing the designated reps with each side. So if the workout calls for 10 reps, you're actually doing 10 per arm, or 20 total reps per set.

## ✳ Split stance

Stand with your right leg in front of your left when pulling with your left arm, and the opposite when pulling with your right. This version will be slightly easier for beginners, and allow heavier weights for more advanced lifters.

## ✳ Tall kneeling

It's exactly the same as the standing version, except you're on your knees, which makes it slightly harder to maintain your balance. I like it more as a core-training exercise than one to develop the upper-back muscles.

## ✳ Half-kneeling

This is a personal favorite for two reasons: The half-kneeling position (you rest on your left knee when you pull with your left arm, and vice versa) is more stable than standing or tall kneeling, which means you can use heavier weights. And the heavier the weight, the tougher the challenge to your core to prevent torso rotation. So you're building more upper-back muscle in tandem with anti-rotational core strength.

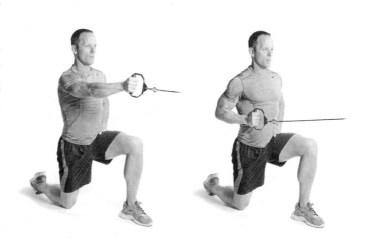

## ✳ Single-leg

Stand on your right leg to pull with your left arm, and on your left to pull with your right. The balance component prevents you from using heavy weights, but it's a fun and challenging exercise to use from time to time with higher reps. It also activates your glutes and hamstrings, since you're leaning forward at the start of the exercise, and then straightening yourself at the end.

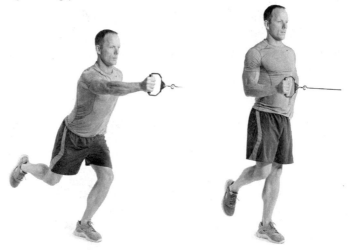

### LEVEL 2

## ✳ Kneeling lat pulldown

**BEST FOR:** basic vertical pulling (although some of the variations create an angle of pull in between vertical and horizontal). Unless and until you're ready for chin-ups and pull-ups, you really can't go wrong with this exercise. And even if you can knock out sets of chin-ups, few of us are strong enough to do them for high reps. Aside from helping you develop strength and size in your upper back and biceps, pulldowns also have an underrated role in helping you develop and maintain full range of movement with your shoulder blades.

**GET READY**

- If you have access to a cable machine with dual, independent pulleys, use those, with a stirrup handle attached to each. For a conventional lat-pulldown station, attach a long bar to the overhead cable apparatus.
- Grab the bar overhand with a grip that's about one and a half times shoulder width (the same width you would use for a barbell bench press, if you do them).

- Kneel in front of the weight stack, pulling the bar down with you so your arms are fully extended overhead.

**MOVE**

- Pull the bar down to your upper chest, *while pushing your chest out to meet the bar.* This will help you keep your shoulder blades down while also pulling them together in back.

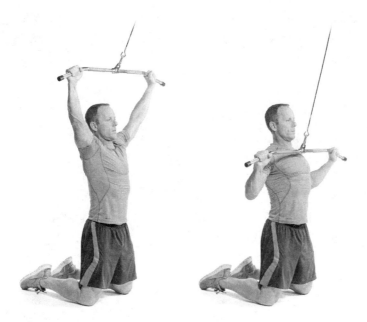

## For More Biceps Work

Use the overhand grip for at least one complete program. After that, you can switch to a shoulder-width, underhand grip to get your biceps more engaged. The triangle handle, which puts your hands a few inches apart with your palms facing each other (aka neutral grip), is an option for yet another program. It puts your arms in their strongest position, allowing you to use a heavier weight. You also get more assistance from your chest muscles than you would with a wider grip.

## SUPERCHARGE IT!

These three variations add a core challenge:

### ✳ Single-arm, half-kneeling

Attach a stirrup handle to the cable pulley. Kneel on your left knee when pulling with your left arm, and vice versa. Remember that you're doing all the designated reps with each side, so for a set of 10 reps you're actually doing 20.

### ✳ Two arms, half-kneeling

Attach a straight bar to the cable pulley, and make sure you do the same number of reps with each leg forward. So if you're doing 2 sets of 15, you can do one set each way. If you're doing an odd number of sets, you can switch legs halfway through the final set.

### ✳ Standing

You can stand with your feet parallel to each other or split apart. If you do the latter, make sure you do equal reps with each leg forward. You can use a straight bar with a wide overhand grip or the triangle handle with a neutral grip.

### LEVEL 3, OPTION 1

### ✳ Dumbbell two-point row

**BEST FOR:** This exercise has appeared in all five NROL books, for good reason. It's a terrific way to work your upper-back muscles while also challenging your core to support your lower back in a bent-over position. The one downside is that your lower back eventually becomes a limiting factor. The most advanced readers will be able to use 50 to 100 percent more weight with the next variation, the three-point row. Still, less advanced lifters should use the two-point row for at least one program in Basic Training or Hypertrophy. The strength and stability you develop will make you better at just about every lift in the program. Use the two-point row for as long as you can increase the weight from one workout to the next, or until you're ready to move up to Level 4. If your strength stalls, or if you feel strain on your back when you use heavier weights, move on to the three-point row.

**GET READY**

- Grab a dumbbell with your nondominant hand. Stand with your feet shoulder-width apart and knees bent slightly.
- Push your hips back as you bend your torso forward.
- Hold the weight straight down from your shoulder with an overhand grip (palm facing back).

**MOVE**

- Pull the weight straight up to the side of your abdomen. Lower it to the starting position, finish all your reps, then repeat the set with the other arm.

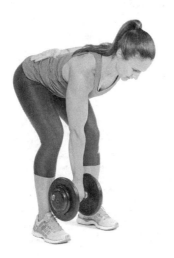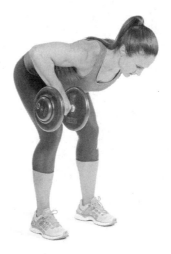

### LEVEL 3, OPTION 2

## ✳ Dumbbell three-point row

**BEST FOR:** lifting heavy weights in any rep range, but especially sets of 10 or fewer. This is one of the best muscle- and strength-building exercises in the book. The simplicity of the exercise allows a short, straight lift with your body in its strongest, most stable position. When you get to this exercise, don't waste it. Use the heaviest weights you can for the prescribed reps, and don't worry if you fall short every now and then.

**GET READY**

- Grab a dumbbell and stand facing a bench or step. As with the single-arm bench press described in Chapter 10, I've found that I do better with this exercise when I start with the dominant hand (your right if you're right-handed), work to exhaustion, and then work even harder to match the reps with the nondominant hand.
- Bend forward at the hips so your torso is parallel to the floor and rest your non-working hand on the bench, while holding the dumbbell straight down from your shoulder.
- Set your shoulders square to the floor, and tighten your torso and hips so you have a stable base for the pull.

**MOVE**

- Pull the weight straight up to the side of your abdomen.
- Lower it to the starting position, finish all your reps, then repeat the set with the other arm.

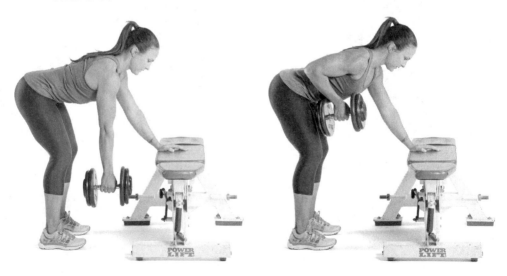

**LEVEL 3, OPTION 3**

## ✳ Dumbbell chest-supported row

**BEST FOR:** relatively inexperienced lifters who feel more comfortable with the extra support. It tends to work better for men than for women, for the obvious reason. It's also difficult to perform with heavier weights because the bigger dumbbells will bang against the edge of the bench at the top of the lift.

**GET READY**

- Set a bench to a 45-degree incline. Grab a pair of dumbbells and lie chest-down, with your head and shoulders beyond the top of the bench, your arms hanging straight down, and your toes on the floor.
- You can turn your palms so they face out (underhand), back (overhand), or toward each other (neutral).

**MOVE**

- Pull the weights to the sides of your torso if you're using a neutral or underhand grip, or to the sides of your chest if you're using an overhand grip with your elbows out.

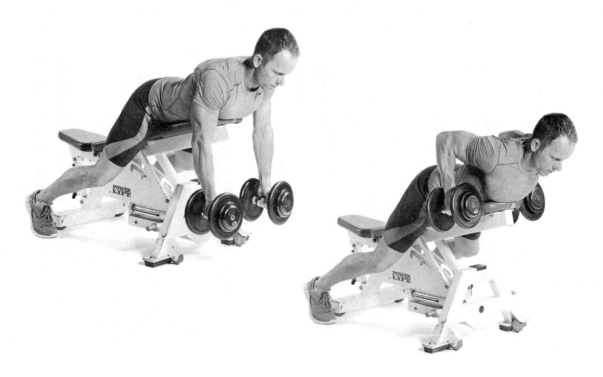

## LEVEL 4

## ✴ Inverted row

**BEST FOR:** everyone; as soon as you're strong enough to do the reps required in any program in Basic Training or Hypertrophy, have at it. This is a great exercise, and with the right setup, it's astoundingly versatile (especially if you can do the suspended variations shown on the next few pages). You can raise the bar to make it easier for higher-rep sets, and lower the bar to make it harder.

### GET READY

- Set up a barbell in a rack so it's somewhere between the height of your waist and hips. (You can also use a Smith machine for this, if you train in a gym that has one.)
- Slide under the bar and grab it overhand, with your hands about one and a half times shoulder width. Set your body in a straight line from neck to ankles, and hang with your arms straight. Only your heels should touch the floor.

### MOVE

- Pull your chest to the bar, return to the starting position, and repeat.
- If you can't get all the reps in your current phase, raise the bar a few inches, which will make it a little easier.

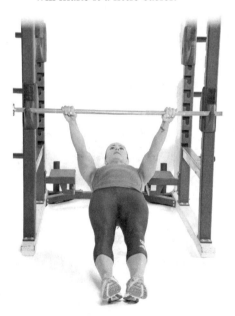 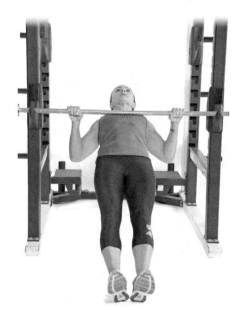

- You can also get more reps by moving your feet a little closer to your torso, with a slight knee bend.

## For More Biceps Work

Use the overhand grip for at least one complete program. After that, you can switch to a shoulder-width, underhand grip for more biceps work.

### SUPERCHARGE IT!

You can only lower the bar so far before your head hits the floor. That's when you can bust out some fun variations: lift one leg, or set both feet on a bench or Swiss ball. When both feet are raised, your shoulders will end up lower than your feet, giving you a new and uniquely challenging angle.

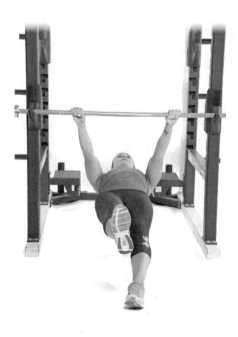
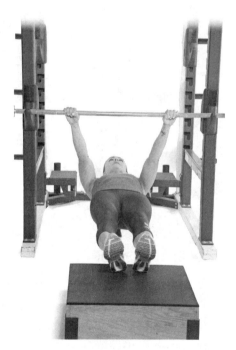

### And If Those Aren't Hard Enough . . .

You can do all the inverted-row variations shown here with a suspension trainer. These are different from the suspended-row variations shown on the following pages, since your shoulders will be directly under the point of attachment.

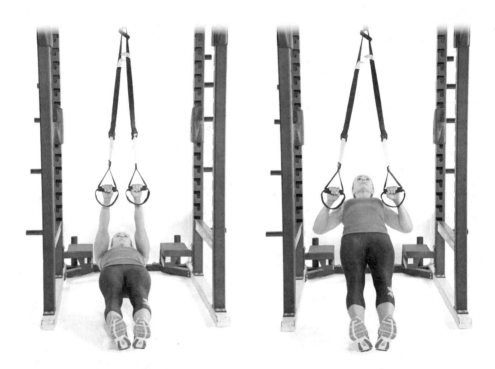

#### LEVEL 4.5

### ✳ Suspended row

**BEST FOR:** It's easiest to explain the benefits of these rows by starting with what they're not. They're not pure muscle- or strength-building exercises. For those, you need the most stable position possible, and the shortest, simplest line of resistance, allowing you to use the heaviest weights you can manage. These angled pulls, using your body weight for resistance, require lots of work from lots of muscles to keep your body stabilized. The range of motion is rarely short and never simple. That's why these exercises are best for intermediate to advanced lifters who can perform complex, unbalanced exercises for 10 or more reps per set. If you qualify (and if you also have a suspension trainer and a place to use it), you'll find these are some of the best exercises for Basic Training and Hypertrophy. The effort they take burns up energy and contributes to the metabolic cost of each workout, leaving you leaner. The complexity of the exercises helps improve your balance, coordination, athleticism, muscular endurance, and overall conditioning, on top of the boost to your strength, muscle size, and core stability.

I'll start by describing the basic version of the exercise, and then show the variations Alwyn uses, ranked by how hard his coauthor finds them.

### GET READY

- Attach the suspension system to something high and sturdy, like a chin-up bar.
- Grab the handles and, facing the attachment point, walk out a couple of steps until the straps are diagonal to the floor.
- Lean back on your heels until your body is diagonal to the floor, with your arms extended and aligned with the straps. Your body should form a straight line from ankles to neck.

### MOVE

- Pull the handles to your sides as you raise yourself to an upright position. Push your chest out to finish the movement.
- Return to the starting position and repeat.

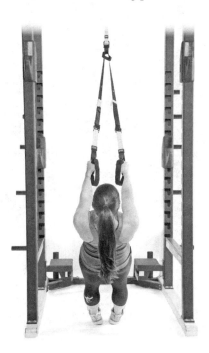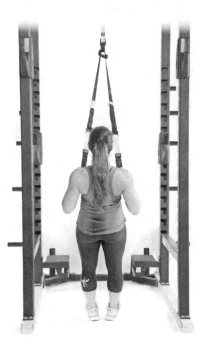

- You can make it harder by walking your heels in closer to the attachment point, which puts your body at a more severe angle, or make it easier by starting with your feet farther away and your body more upright.

**SUPERCHARGE IT!**

## ✴ Suspended single-arm row

Same thing, only with one arm at a time, holding both handles in one hand. (Do all the designated reps with each arm.) Your body will have to work hard to resist rotation. This is an advanced version of the Level 1 standing cable row.

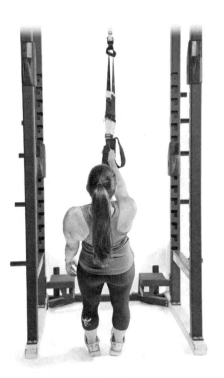 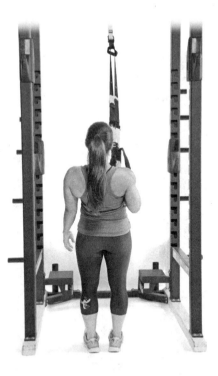

## ✳ Suspended single-arm row with rotation

- Set up with both feet on the floor, leaning back, with both handles in your right hand. But this time start with your arm bent and the handles at your chest, and your left arm extended in front of you, aligned with the straps.
- Reach back with your left arm and rotate to your left as you extend your right arm.
- Rotate back to your right as you pull the handles to your chest with your right arm.
- Do all your reps, switch sides, and repeat.
- You'll see the exercise on YouTube videos with knees bent (sometimes with hips bent as well, turning it into a hybrid squat with rotation), but Alwyn prefers that you keep your body in a straight line from ankles to neck.

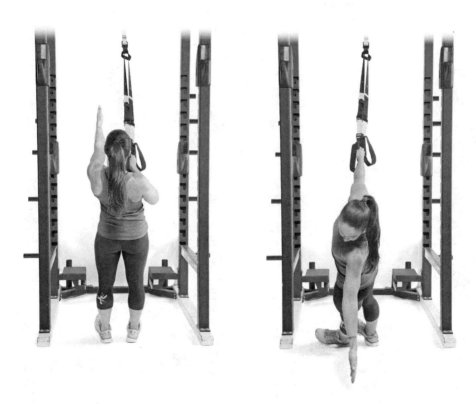

**LEVEL 5**

★ **Chin-up**

**BEST FOR:** pure strength and size for those who can do the designated number of reps for any of these programs. It's the best exercise most of us do for our lats and biceps.

**GET READY**

- Grab the chin-up bar with a shoulder-width, underhand grip, and hang from the bar with your knees bent and ankles crossed behind you. Your body should form a straight line from neck to knees.

**MOVE**

- Pull your chest up to the bar, lower yourself, and repeat.

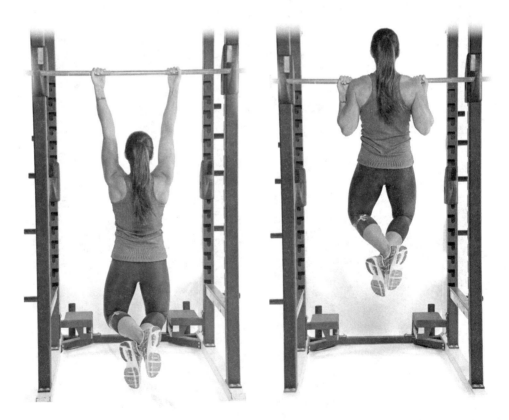

## SUPERCHARGE IT!

Weighted chins, using a dipping belt with a dumbbell or weight plate attached, are a terrific choice for the Strength & Power programs, since you can easily add and subtract weight.

## High-Rep Alternative

Attach a resistance band to the chin-up bar, and loop it around your knees. You should be able to get several more reps per set, making it a viable choice for Hypertrophy.

## And If Your Shoulders Can Handle It . . .

Consider the pull-up, in which you use an overhand grip with your hands just outside shoulder width.

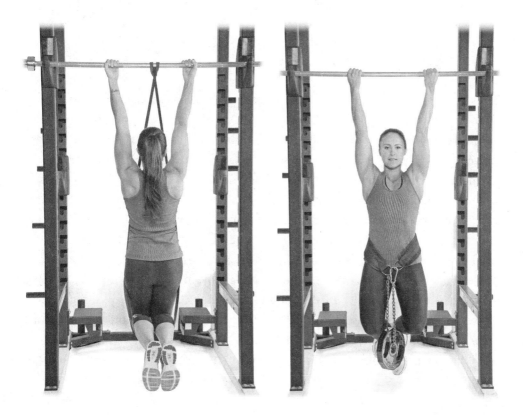

12

# Lunge

THERE'S AN EASY WAY TO DISTINGUISH lunges from similar exercises in the single-leg-stance category in Chapter 13: With a lunge, the targeted muscles work with both feet on the floor, a bench, or a step. You may step backward (reverse lunge) or forward (traveling lunge), but both feet are on something solid during the parts of the exercise in which you're lowering or raising your body.

Your front knee will always be bent at least 90 degrees on lunges, with your torso as upright as possible, minimizing action at your hip joints. That's why many coaches refer to the lunge as a "knee-dominant" or "quad-dominant" exercise. But, as Alwyn and I have stressed throughout the NROL series, looking at any exercise in terms of a single joint or set of muscles sells it short. It's the movement pattern that matters, and the lunge is a movement you use in sports, hiking or climbing, or pushing a lawn-mower or wheelbarrow up a slope. If the activity includes one leg out in front of the other, the lunge can help you do it better.

Which is not to play down muscle development. A basic split squat—a lunge without the part where you actually lunge forward or back—works the quadriceps as thoroughly as you want to work them. Put a barbell on your shoulders, as you would for a front or back squat, stand with one foot in front of the other, drop into the lunge position, and rise back up. Only your strength and ambition limit the amount of weight you can use.

Of course the quadriceps don't operate in isolation. The hamstrings and glutes work to straighten your hip. Muscles in your inner thighs (adductors) and outer hips (abductors) work to keep you balanced. When there's movement involved, whether it's forward or backward, your lower-leg muscles come into play. (I noted in *NROL for Life* that my calves seem to get bigger when I do reverse lunges from a step, one of the Level 2 variations.)

Then you have a range of possibilities for core development. I'm a huge believer in doing exercises with an offset load, usually holding a single dumbbell or kettlebell to one side, and then letting your body figure out how to keep you upright. If the load is on your left side—that is, you're holding a dumbbell with your left hand, either at your side, at your shoulder, or overhead—you'll call into action the quadratus lumborum on your right side. The QL muscle originates on the top of your pelvis and inserts in several places along your bottom rib and the outer edges of your lumbar vertebrae. The textbook description says that the QL on your right side pulls you upright when you're bent over to your left. But given how unimportant that action is, and given the fact that your internal and external oblique muscles help perform it, it makes sense that the QL is most often employed in preventing the movement in the first place. When we talk about core muscles "keeping your lower back and pelvis in a safe, neutral position," this is what we mean.

Thus, the lunge offers a range of possibilities for training. For pure strength and muscle development, you can load it up with heavy weights for low or medium reps in the Hypertrophy programs. In Basic Training, with high reps, lunge variations give you a hellacious metabolic beatdown. An unbalanced load develops core stability in either type of program. That's in addition to the challenges to your mobility and coordination, which inevitably come as a shock to me when I return to one of these exercises after a long respite.

## LEVEL 1
### ✳ Split squat

**BEST FOR:** whatever you want it to be. Everyone should start with this exercise for at least one workout. And no one should use an external load until you know you can do 15 good reps with each leg with just your body weight. If you can't, then do body-weight split squats as shown here until you can, or until you finish Basic Training I, whichever comes first. If you're sure you can do 15, then do that as a warm-up set, and choose a form of resistance for your work sets. You can use anything you see in this chapter: dumbbells, barbell, one or two kettlebells. Just do the basic split squat for at least one workout before you move on to the higher-level lunges.

**GET READY**

- Stand with your hands behind your head in the prisoner grip and your feet hip-width apart. Take a long step back with your right leg. This is your starting position.

**MOVE**

- Lower yourself until the top of your left thigh is parallel to the floor and your right knee nearly touches the floor.
- Return to the starting position and repeat until you finish all your reps. Switch legs and repeat the same number of reps. That's one set.

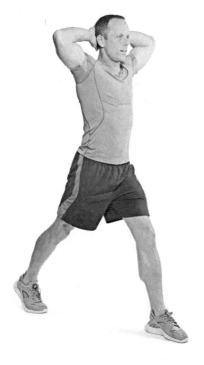
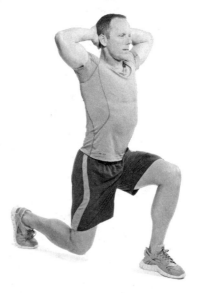

## LEVEL 2

### ✳ Reverse lunge

**BEST FOR:** everything you want to accomplish in the weight room. For inexperienced lifters, it's a simple and easy progression from the split squat. (You should do it holding dumbbells, as shown here, before trying any of the more advanced variations.) For those of us with creaky knees, it allows the highest-quality work with the least discomfort. And for the most advanced and confident lifters, you have a world of options, only a few of which are shown here. You can exercise your imagination along with your muscles. Anything you can lift and hold can be an effective form of resistance.

**GET READY**

- Grab a pair of dumbbells and stand holding them at your sides, with your feet hip-width apart.

**MOVE**

- Take a long step back with your right foot and lower yourself until the top of your left thigh is parallel to the floor and your right knee nearly touches the floor. Keep your torso upright.
- Step back to the starting position and repeat until you finish all your reps. Switch legs and repeat. That's one set.

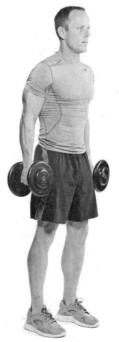
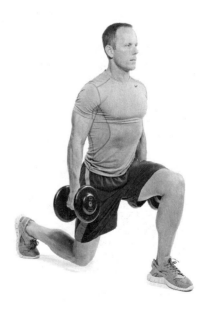

SUPERCHARGE IT!

# ✳ Reverse lunge from step

One of my personal favorites: Start with both feet on a box or step that's about 6 inches high. Step back with your right foot and lower yourself into a deeper lunge. Your left thigh will end up below parallel to the floor. The extra range of motion should provide an extra muscle-building stimulus, but it also comes with increased risk to your upper-thigh and lower-abdominal tissues. Start cautiously and add weight in small increments.

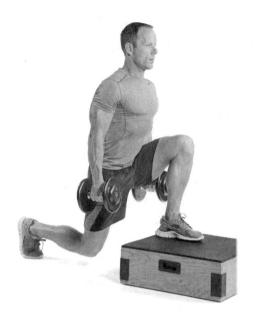

# ✳ Goblet reverse lunge

Hold a dumbbell, kettlebell, or weight plate against your chest. The goblet lunge makes it easier to get through a high-rep set, since your grip strength won't be as much of a limiting factor as it would be holding dumbbells at your sides. Even if the resistance is the same or less than you'd use with dumbbells, it's a slightly harder exercise because the center of gravity is higher.

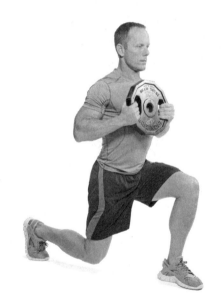

## ✴ Barbell reverse lunge

You can hold the barbell behind your shoulders, as you would for a back squat (shown on pages 88–89), or in the front-squat position, as shown here. It's a new exercise for me, and the combination of a higher center of gravity with a heavy load makes it a fun challenge.

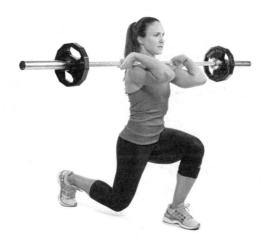

## ✴ Overhead reverse lunge

We show it here with a barbell, but you can hold two dumbbells or a single weight plate overhead.

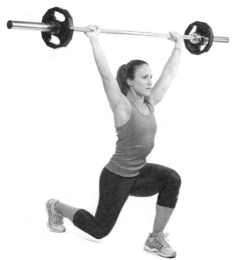

### ✳ Offset reverse lunge

You want to hold the weight on the same side as the working leg. If you're stepping back with your right leg, your left leg is the one that's doing the lifting. That means you hold the weight in your left hand. You can hold a single dumbbell at shoulder level, or a single kettlebell in the rack position.

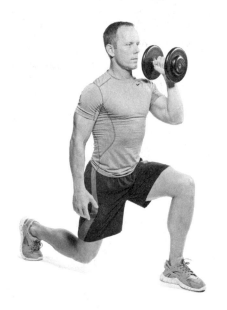

### ✳ Overhead offset reverse lunge from step

You can see where this is going. Advanced lifters can mix and match any or all of these variations. One switch: When you're holding an offset weight overhead, you probably want to hold it opposite the working leg. Thus, if you're stepping back with your right leg, you hold the weight overhead with your right hand.

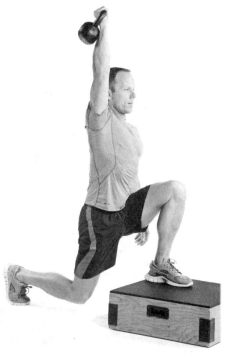

**LEVEL 2.5**

✳ **Side lunge**

**BEST FOR:** well-balanced lower-body muscle development, especially for athletes in sports that include a lot of lateral movement. It's not a primary training exercise, but it's a variation you can use for a single program in Basic Training or Hypertrophy. You'll hit the adductors (inner-thigh muscles) especially hard.

**GET READY**

- Grab a dumbbell or kettlebell and hold it with both hands in front of your chest, as you would for a goblet squat.
- Stand with your feet shoulder-width apart, toes pointed forward.

**MOVE**

- Take a long step to your left, push your hips back, and drop into a deep squat, with your left thigh parallel to the floor. Your left knee will be aligned with your left foot, while your right leg remains straight. Both feet are flat on the floor. Your torso will lean forward slightly from the hips, but without bending or twisting to either side.
- Push back up to the starting position.
- You can do all your reps to the left, then switch sides and repeat, or alternate sides.
- Your shoulders and hips will face forward and remain aligned with each other throughout the movement.

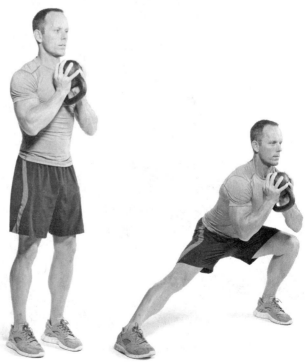

# ✳ Split squat, rear foot elevated

**BEST FOR:** pure muscle development, mainly focused on the quadriceps. It's not an easy or fun exercise, but it does the job.

### GET READY

- You can hold dumbbells at your sides or a single dumbbell, kettlebell, or weight plate against your chest in the goblet-squat position.
- Set the toes of your right foot on a low step, 6 to 8 inches high, and get into split-squat position by taking a long step forward with your left foot.

### MOVE

- Lower yourself until the top of your left thigh is parallel to the floor, keeping your torso upright.
- Push back to the starting position, and do all your reps before switching legs and repeating.

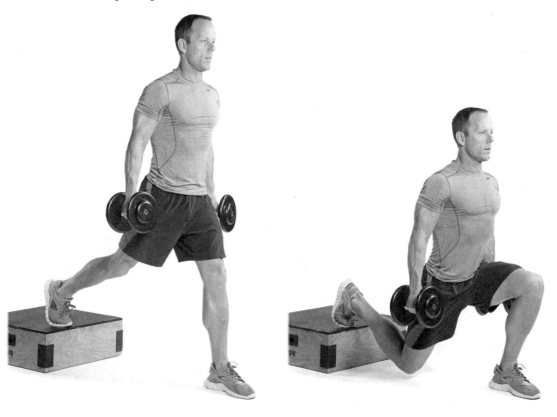

## SUPERCHARGE IT!

## ✴ Bulgarian split squat

Same thing, only with the instep of your rear foot resting on a box or bench that's at least 12 inches high. Remember that the entire benefit of the exercise comes from the range of motion. If you raise the elevation of your rear foot but compensate by cutting short the movement with your working leg, you haven't really accomplished anything. It's supposed to be brutal, and you're supposed to hate it.

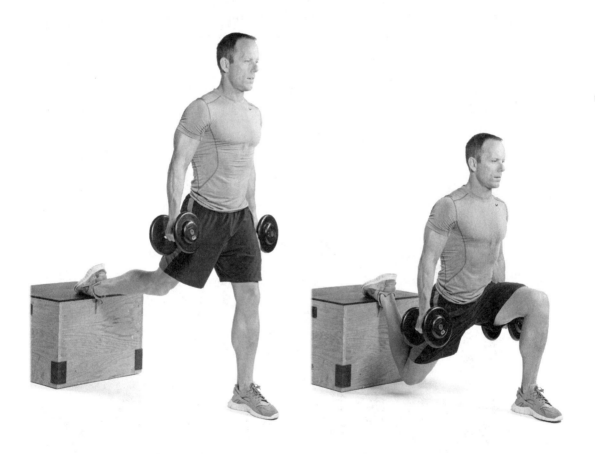

## ✳ Suspended split squat

With the suspension system attached to an overhead support, turn your back to the straps and put your right foot into the loops. Hop forward with your left foot until you're in a comfortable position for split squats. Drop down into the lunge position and push back up. (You may want to put a pad beneath your right knee, both to protect it and to give you a sense of how low to go for a full range of motion.) Do your reps, switch legs, and repeat.

I like to use my arms in a running motion. With the left leg forward, drive your right arm up on the descent, and your left arm up as you rise. When your right leg is forward, drive with your left arm on the descent. You can hold a pair of light dumbbells as you do it.

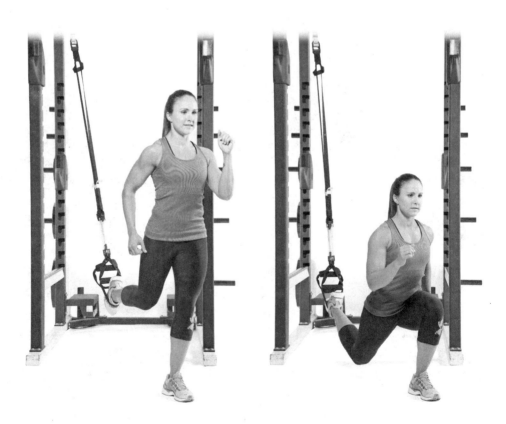

## LEVEL 4

## ✳ Forward lunge

**BEST FOR:** advanced-level lifters who can do it without any knee discomfort or pain. Why advanced? Haven't beginners been doing forward lunges as long as people have done exercise at all? And isn't the forward lunge really just a *lunge*, as in, the only exercise in this chapter that meets the dictionary definition of the word? Yes, but Alwyn doesn't care. He doesn't want you to do this exercise until you've worked your way up through Level 2 (using multiple variations) and Level 3. That means you'll probably be in Hypertrophy II or III by the time you get to the forward lunge, by which time you'll need to use a relatively heavy resistance for low-rep sets.

### GET READY
- Choose a form of resistance, which can be anything you've seen so far in this chapter: dumbbells, kettlebells, or a barbell (as shown).
- Stand with your feet hip-width apart.

### MOVE
- Take a long step forward with your left leg, and lower yourself until the top of your left thigh is parallel to the floor. Your right knee should almost touch the floor while your torso remains upright.
- Push back to the starting position.
- Repeat with your right leg, and alternate until you've done all the repetitions with each leg.

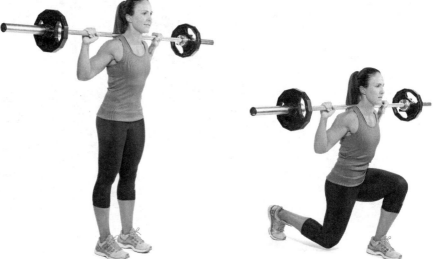

## SUPERCHARGE IT!

You can do anything you've seen so far in this chapter: offset load, overhead, overhead offset . . . Just make sure you've done conventional forward lunges with relatively heavy resistance for at least one program. Now here's one of my favorite variations:

## ✴ Forward lunge to step

Stand 2 to 3 feet behind a low step (6 to 8 inches high). Step forward with your left leg and set your left foot on the step. Drop into a deep lunge, then push back to the starting position. Repeat with your right leg.

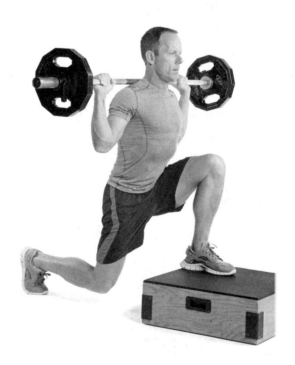

## LEVEL 5
### ✳ Walking lunge

**BEST FOR:** In *NROL for Life*, I wrote this: "I scratch my head when I see this exercise used in entry-level workout programs. I've always considered it an advanced lunge variation—one I rarely do in my own workouts—and Alwyn agrees. This is the first time he's included it in the NROL series, even though we've featured some extraordinarily challenging (dare I say "badass"?) exercises." A trainer friend told me he finds it easier both for himself and his clients than our Level 4 exercise, the forward lunge. He said that maintaining forward momentum is easier on the knees than going forward, braking, and pushing back. It's a valid point, but it doesn't change Alwyn's rationale for putting this one after the traditional lunge. He wants *you* to be advanced before you use it in your workouts. You'll be able to use heavier weights with better form, and get more out of it. Personally, for what it's worth, I don't do many forward or walking lunges at all, just because I never really get bored with the Level 2 and 3 exercises, or feel that I've maxed out on them.

**GET READY**

- Grab a pair of dumbbells (probably the most popular form of resistance for walking lunges; you can use a barbell, but it seems too hard-core even for a book with "Supercharged" in the title), and stand holding them at your sides with your feet hip-width apart.

**MOVE**

- Take a long step forward with your left leg, as described previously.
- Push off your right foot and step forward into a lunge with your right leg.
- Continue lunging forward, alternating legs, until you've done all the repetitions with each leg.

# 13

# Single-Leg Stance

THIS IS THE BOOK'S HYBRID CATEGORY, with exercises distinguished by a technicality, rather than a specific movement pattern or muscle action. You perform them with one foot on a solid surface, and that leg does all the work. That's different from the lunges in Chapter 12, in which both feet are grounded at the time of the lift.

The muscles you use will vary. Step-ups, single-leg Romanian deadlifts, and single-leg deadlifts are considered hip-dominant exercises, meaning your glutes and hamstrings are the prime movers. Single-leg squats, like lunges, are typically placed in the knee- or quad-dominant category.

I don't think your body will agree.

Take the step-up, the Level 1 exercise. For it to be a hip-dominant exercise, you have to remember to push down with the heel of your working leg—the one that's planted on a box or step—to activate your hamstrings and glutes. Inexperienced lifters will almost always push off the ball of the foot, and get more of the quadriceps involved (especially the vastus medialis, the part of the muscle just above the inside half of the knee). That's assuming you only push off on one leg to begin with. The more tired you get, the more likely you are to push off the floor with the leg that isn't supposed to work at all. It's just along for the ride.

Then you have the single-leg Romanian deadlift at Level 3. If you aren't used to it, it becomes a coordination challenge, one you'll feel in your weakest link. It might be the foot and ankle of your working leg, it might be your lower back, or it might even be your shoulders, if you struggle to stabilize your upper back when you're bent forward. It's unlikely that you'll feel it in your glutes and hamstrings the first time you try it . . . unless overly tight hamstrings are your weakest link. Then you'll feel the heck out of it.

Finally, in Levels 4 and 5 you have the single-leg squat and deadlift. For me, they're both knee-dominant exercises, but not in a good way. (Maybe I should call them knee-dominatrix.) I think most readers will experience them as core-dominant exercises. These exercises will find and expose any part of your core that isn't up to factory standards.

The great thing about these exercises is that they correct the problems they identify, as long as you use them with appropriate caution. Master each level before moving up to the next, and when you get stuck, feel free to stay at that level for multiple programs until your body figures it out.

And if you reach a level where the exercise just hurts, with no discernible benefit, simply acknowledge that it's not for you. There's plenty to do in Levels 1, 2, and 3. You don't need to injure yourself for the temporary satisfaction of saying you've mastered an advanced exercise.

## LEVEL 1

✳ ## Step-up

**BEST FOR:** everyone, in any program in Basic Training or Hypertrophy. I'm still figuring out new ways to challenge myself with step-ups.

### GET READY

- First you have to find a step, box, or bench to step up onto. Or, if you have choices, decide how high a step you can handle. For lifters with knee problems like mine, I recommend a low step: 8 to 12 inches. Healthy and ambitious lifters can start higher.
- Grab a pair of dumbbells and hold them at arm's length at your sides. Remember that you have to hold the weights long enough to complete the repetitions. In Basic Training I, that's 15 reps with each leg.
- Place your left foot flat on the step, with your right foot on the floor.

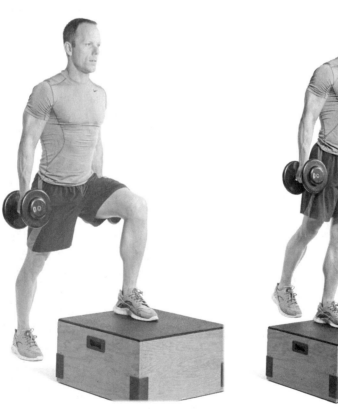
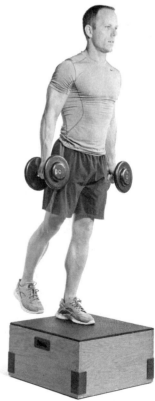

**MOVE**

- Push down through the heel of your left foot and lift yourself up so your right leg is even with your left.
- Brush the step with your right foot to complete the repetition, but don't rest it on the step. You want to keep the tension on the working muscles of your left leg.
- Lower your right foot to the floor.
- Do all your reps with your left leg, then repeat with your right.

**SUPERCHARGE IT!**

# ✳ Barbell step-up

Hold a barbell as you would for the back squat shown on pages 88–89. You can really load this one up, making it a great choice for the Hypertrophy programs. It also addresses the major drawback of the traditional step-up with dumbbells, which is that your grip may give out before you fully exhaust your leg muscles. The barbell version can relieve that problem, although it's not for everyone. It's a challenge to your strength, balance, skill, and confidence. One time when I was using what for me was a heavy load, I had to stop between sets to ask a young woman not to preen in the mirror while I lifted. "You *really* don't want me to lose my focus with that much weight on my shoulders," I told her. (I never saw her again, which is probably best for everyone.)

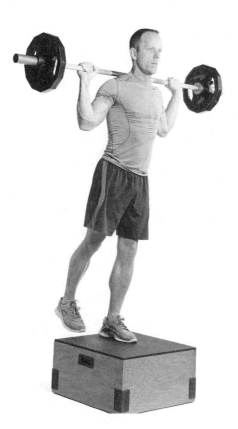

### ✳ Sprinter step-up

To make the exercise faster and more fatiguing, push down hard with your working leg, and bring the knee of the nonworking leg up toward your chest. Once you've gotten the hang of it, bring the knee up explosively.

### LEVEL 2

### ✳ Offset-loaded step-up

**BEST FOR:** This is a simple but important progression, adding a stability challenge to the basic step-up. You should be able to use a challenging weight, since you're holding the weight in only one hand at a time.

**GET READY/MOVE**

- Grab a dumbbell or kettlebell with your left hand and hold it at arm's length on your left side.
- Place your left foot on the step, and follow the steps described earlier.
- Do all your reps, switch the weight to your right hand, and repeat with your right leg.

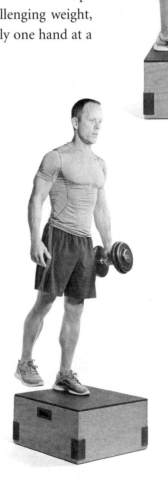

## SUPERCHARGE IT!

Hold a single dumbbell alongside your shoulder, or a single kettlebell in the rack position. As before, hold it in your left hand when stepping up with your left leg, and vice versa.

## TURBOCHARGE IT!

Not ambitious enough for you? Hold a single dumbbell or kettlebell overhead in your right hand while stepping up with your left leg. Be cautious with the weight on this one (although, as Alwyn notes, it won't take long to figure out if you started too heavy).

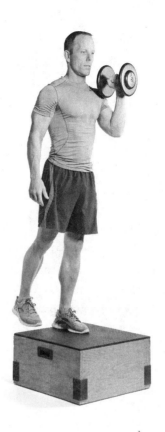

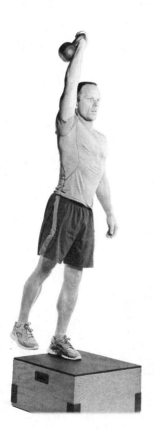

### LEVEL 2.25

## ✳ Crossover step-up

**BEST FOR:** a combined core and lateral-movement challenge for experienced lifters. Try it for one program in Basic Training or Hypertrophy.

### GET READY

- Hold a heavy dumbbell in your right hand and stand next to a bench or step, with your left leg closer to the step and about 12 inches away. (Taller lifters should stand farther away, and shorter lifters may need to get closer.)

### MOVE

- Cross your right leg in front of your left and plant your right foot on the step.
- Push yourself up to the step, without touching it with your left foot.
- Step down with your left foot, followed by your right.
- Do all your reps, and then switch sides.
- After your first set, stand farther away from the step on subsequent sets.

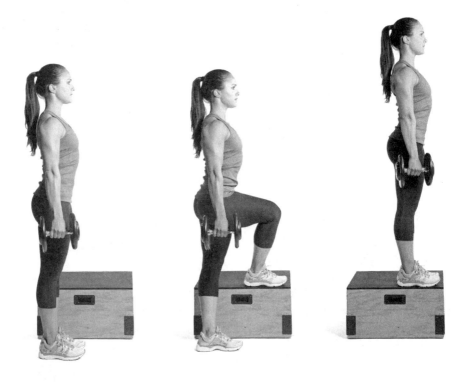

**LEVEL 2.75**

## ✳ Overhead step-up

**BEST FOR:** a total-body challenge for advanced lifters in Basic Training or Hypertrophy.

**GET READY**

- Grab a light barbell (for men, I recommend starting with just the 45-pound Olympic bar; for women, try a 10-pound standard bar), a pair of dumbbells or kettlebells, a weight plate, or anything else you can hold overhead.
- Set your left foot on the step with the weight overhead.

**MOVE**

- Push down through the heel of your left foot and lift yourself up so your right leg is even with your left.
- Brush the step with your right foot, then lower it to the floor.
- Do all your reps with your left leg.
- You'll probably want to set the weight down and catch your breath before you pick it up again and repeat the set with your right leg.

### SUPERCHARGE IT!

Try the overhead sprinter step-up: Holding the weight overhead, bring the knee of your nonworking leg up toward your chest on each repetition.

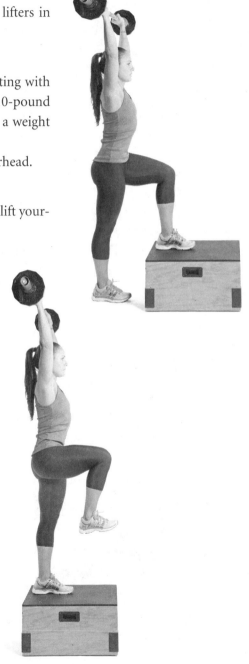

## LEVEL 3

# ✳ Single-leg Romanian deadlift

**BEST FOR:** Alwyn has used this exercise in every book since *NROL for Women*, and it's one all readers should work up to by Hypertrophy III. It's a balance challenge, a core challenge, and a pure muscle builder for your glutes and hamstrings.

**GET READY**

- Grab a dumbbell with your right hand and hold it at arm's length at your side as you stand with your feet together.

**MOVE**

- Hinge at the hip as you bend your torso toward the floor and extend your right leg behind you.
- Lower the weight toward the floor, with your right arm hanging straight down from your shoulder. Your right arm and left leg should be perpendicular to the floor. Do whatever you need to do with your left arm for balance.
- Your neck, torso, and right leg should form a straight line, with your hips and shoulders square to the floor. If you have great balance and range of motion, that line will be parallel to the floor; don't worry if you can't get there right away. The key is to form that straight line.
- Return to the starting position, trying not to put weight on your right leg, and do all your reps. Remember that your left leg is working, even though your right leg is moving. You want to feel the contraction in your left glute.
- Repeat the set with your right leg, holding the weight in your left hand.

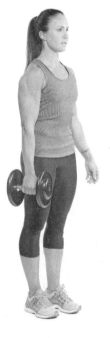

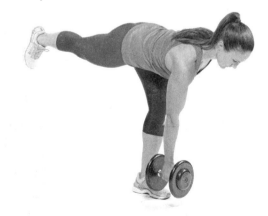

## LEVEL 4

## ✳ Single-leg squat

**BEST FOR:** intermediate to advanced lifters who have used Levels 1 to 3 successfully. The key to this exercise is to remember that each of us will have a different range of motion, for different reasons. The issue might be core stability, the strength of supporting muscles in your inner and outer thighs, hip mobility, or the integrity of your knee joints.

### GET READY

- You'll need a box or step that's at least 12 inches high and a light dumbbell or kettlebell to hold in both hands as a counterbalance.
- Stand on your left foot near the right edge of the box, with your right foot even with your left but hanging out in space over the side of the box.
- Hold the weight in both hands.

### MOVE

- Extend your arms in front of you as you push your hips back and lower yourself as far as you can go, allowing your left knee to bend naturally as your right foot goes below the edge of the box and your right leg extends forward.
- Push back up to the starting position, finish your reps with your left leg, switch sides, and repeat the set.
- In subsequent workouts, the goal is to increase reps and range of motion, rather than add to the weight you're using as a counterbalance.

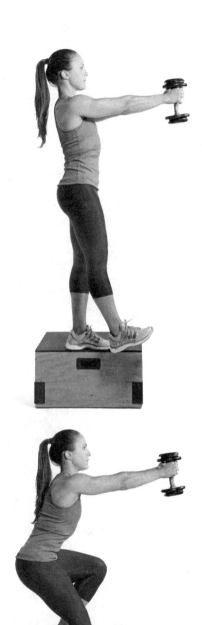

**USEFUL ALTERNATIVES**

## ✴ Supported single-leg squat

If you have a TRX or similar suspension system, this one is easier to perform, especially for higher reps. Take a light grip on the handles, stand facing the attachment point, lift your nonworking leg, push your hips back, and lower yourself as far as you can. Lift back up to the starting position. Try to rely less on the straps over time.

## ✴ Pistol squat

Hold a kettlebell or dumbbell in front of you with both hands. Lift your non-working leg off the floor. Push your hips back as you extend your arms and your nonworking leg forward. Descend as far as you can, then push back up. Keep in mind that very few people can attain the range of motion shown by our model in these photos.

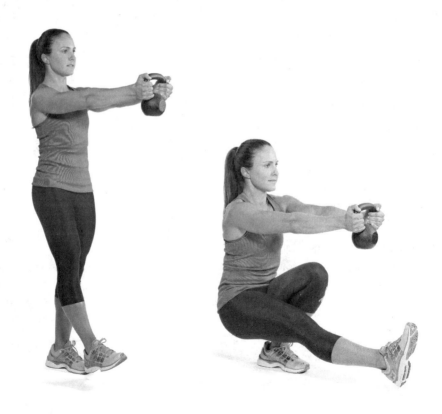

**LEVEL 5**

## ✳ Single-leg deadlift

**BEST FOR:** advanced lifters who're ready to do a single-leg movement with challenging weights. This is one of those exercises where the line between "squat" and "deadlift" blurs to the point of nonexistence. The weights are at arm's length, but you aren't lifting them off the floor. Your torso is bent farther forward, but there isn't really much difference in muscle activation. There's probably more work for your glutes and less for your quadriceps, but only at the margins. The real progression here is that you're positioned to use heavier weights.

**GET READY**

- Grab a pair of dumbbells and stand holding them at your sides.
- Lift your right foot off the floor behind you, bending your right knee about 90 degrees while keeping your thighs parallel to each other.

**MOVE**

- Push your hips back and lower yourself as far as you can.
- Try to keep your non-working leg in a similar position, with your thigh perpendicular to the floor and knee bent about 90 degrees.
- Push back up to the starting position, finish all your reps, and repeat with your right leg.

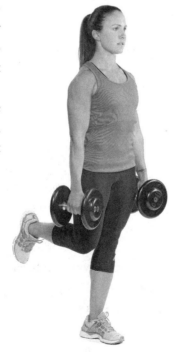
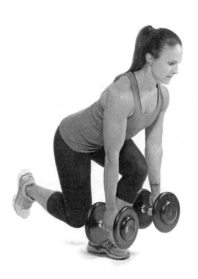

# Core Training

As FITNESS-BOOK AUTHORS, ALWYN AND I like to think of ourselves as the cure for cognitive dissonance. The goal of each book is to present a unified system of exercise and weight management. Problem is, the theory evolves, and we sometimes end up causing as much confusion as we resolve.

Take the crunch, for example.

Alwyn included crunch variations in *NROL* and *NROL for Women*, but with *NROL for Abs* we went in a very different direction with core training. Rather than prescribing exercises that emphasized contraction of the abdominal muscles, Alwyn focused on exercises that *prevent* movement. *Abs* and *Life* include complex core-training programs in which crunches are replaced by progressions that begin with fairly simple stability exercises—planks and side planks—and end with advanced exercises in which multiple limbs are moving while your core remains stabilized.

Alwyn knows it works because he sees his clients' results on a daily basis. I know it works because I hear it from countless readers. Since I test-drove the program several years ago I've never once gone into the gym thinking, "I really miss those crunches." Every now and then I'll test my core strength with an extremely strict sit-up, with my legs straight and flat on the floor, and my arms straight overhead, just to see if I can do it. My arms have to stay next to my ears throughout the movement. If I jerk my arms forward or lift my legs off the floor, I fail.

The last time I failed was the first time I tried it, in 2008, back when I was still doing crunches. I changed my approach to core training soon after, and haven't failed the test since.

My own results are proof of nothing, especially when you consider all the things I *can't* do. But I hope they explain my conviction that a comprehensive core-training program from a coach like Alwyn beats the snot out of a random collection of crunches.

The NROL core-training philosophy goes something like this:

1. The core includes all the muscles that act on the lower back and pelvis: abdominals, spinal erectors, hip flexors, glutes, hamstrings. We also include the lats, as noted in Chapter 2, since those fibers originate along the lower back and top of the pelvis, and thus play a role in stabilizing your spine.

2. The lumbar spine has a small range of motion—a few degrees forward and back, with a tiny ability to rotate. It's safest to train in what we call a neutral position, in which your spine resists movement. This applies to almost every exercise in this book.

3. It's not enough to be cognizant of your lower-back posture while lifting. You should also do specific exercises, like the ones in this chapter, to train your core to remain stabilized.

4. The first goal of stability training is to develop endurance in your core muscles, along with the strength to resist forces that threaten to pull your spine and pelvis out of that neutral zone.

5. For most readers, it won't take long to build a base of core strength and endurance with basic planks and side planks. That's why it's important to advance to higher-level exercises. Those exercises are harder, and develop qualities beyond baseline stability, including balance, coordination, and fatigue resistance. Now you're building true fitness.

6. Meanwhile, you're moving ahead in the other areas of Alwyn's system: mobility, power, strength, metabolic fitness. Core training is now integrated into your total-body fitness program, rather than isolated within it. You'll see that all training is core training, just as all training contributes to mobility, power, strength, and overall conditioning.

7. The lines between different training components may blur, but the results come into sharp focus. You're leaner, stronger, more muscular, more athletic, more active, more fit.

This is why someone doing NROL workouts is going to stand apart from most lifters in most commercial gyms. While others do crunches, repetitively squeezing abdominal muscles with the magical idea that if you make those muscles bigger your waist will somehow get smaller, you'll focus on core stability. While others use machines with the goal of building muscles in isolation, you'll mostly use free weights and your own body weight to build them through coordinated action. While others separate "strength" and "cardio," you'll develop muscular and cardiovascular fitness simultaneously. While others try to outsmart their bodies to indulge a fantasy of having arms or abs or buttocks like the celebrity of the moment, you'll work with your physiology to develop the best shape possible given your genetics, ambition, and ability to stick with your plan.

Is this the only way to train? No, of course not. Every day in the gym I see men and women doing the opposite of Alwyn's style of training. Some of them appear to be in much better shape than me. I'm the last guy to argue that there's only One True Path to fitness. You can find lots of ways to get there. Then again, Alwyn and I don't write these books for lifters who're sold on a dissimilar system because they're satisfied with the results. We write for people who *don't* get what they want from other types of programs, and are ready to try something new. (Along with readers who, like me, are happy with our results from previous NROL programs and want to continue with Alwyn's newest.)

## THE PROGRAM

Alwyn includes three categories of core exercises:

- **Stabilization**, in which nothing moves and the challenge is to hold a static position
- **Dynamic stabilization**, in which one or more limbs move around a stabilized base of support
- **Integrated stabilization** (presented here as Level 5 in the dynamic-stabilization category), in which your entire body moves and your core has to resist multiple challenges to its stability

An important question: What exactly are we stabilizing *against*? Let's start with the end result. Say you're lifting a heavy weight overhead. Bending backward—*spinal extension*—could compress your lumbar discs and possibly lead to injury. So you want to do exercises that train your body to resist spinal extension. Those anti-extension exercises—starting with planks—are as important as any in the program.

Now imagine that you're lifting up an unbalanced load, anything from a sack of dog food to a sleeping toddler. You need your torso to stay upright, which means not bending to the side, an action called *lateral flexion*. The goal of exercises like side planks is to teach your body to resist lateral flexion.

Then there's *rotation*. Of course twisting and turning are important in any sport in which you throw, hit, or catch (or avoid being thrown, hit, or caught). But the discs in your lower back can only twist about 2 degrees. You need to make sure your shoulders turn while your lower back and pelvis remain stable. That's why anti-rotation exercises are a key part of core training.

The other movement you want to resist is *spinal flexion*. For example, if you were doing a squat or a deadlift with a heavy load and your lumbar spine went from its natural arch to a forward bend, the result could be disastrous. This isn't an issue Alwyn addresses with core training so much as one he tries not to make worse with spine-flexing exercises. What are the muscles that flex your spine out of its natural arch? The rectus abdominis (the six-pack muscle) and the obliques. What are the muscles that you make bigger and stronger with sit-ups and crunches? The rectus abdominis and the obliques. In sports and real life, how important is it for your muscles to generate force while bending your torso forward? Not very. (Combat sports are an obvious exception.)

The abdominals are certainly important muscles, and they'll get lots of work in anti-extension, anti-rotation, and anti-lateral flexion exercises. They'll also work to safeguard your back in every movement pattern in Alwyn's workouts, while helping you transfer force from lower body to upper body, and from upper to lower. You just won't work them in ways that might create more problems than they solve.

There's one other type of exercise in this chapter: *hip flexion*. You'll find hip-flexion exercises in the dynamic stabilization category, starting at Level 3. I explain their purpose in the "Hip Ops" sidebar on page 197. For accounting purposes, these are the equivalent of anti-extension exercises.

## PROGRESSION

Here's how you get all you can out of core training:

### 1. Improve your performance on each exercise, each workout.

With the stabilization exercises, you have a time goal (30 seconds for planks, 30 seconds on each side for side planks). If you don't hit that goal the first time you try the exercise, keep working at it until you do.

In dynamic and integrated stabilization, you work with an external load most of the time, so you improve by:

- Perfecting your form
- Doing more reps with your current weight
- Using more weight

### 2. Use more advanced exercises within the category.

You need to move up to more challenging stabilization exercises as soon as you can do one of them for the maximum suggested time. Since it's easier to hold a plank for 30 seconds than it is to hold a side plank for the same time, you'll go through plank variations much faster, and spend more time with each side-plank option.

With dynamic stabilization, you know it's time to advance to the next level when:

- You can't use heavier weights without altering your form.
- You finish your current program.

*You don't want these exercises to be easy.* As soon as an exercise is no longer challenging, you need to move up.

## COME FULL CIRCLE

You'll notice as you work your way through the system that Alwyn has you return to the stabilization category multiple times, even in the Strength & Power programs. This is one of the most important features of his programs, and it's at the heart of his training philosophy: *There's no point in developing a fitness quality if you're just going to abandon it.* Learning and mastering the more advanced exercises in this book is key to getting the results you want. But from time to time you have to return to the basics to make sure your body retains those qualities.

Alwyn and I started working on *NROL for Abs* in 2009, and since then I've embraced the idea of circling back to entry-level exercises. My body *always* feels better after using simple exercises like planks and side planks for a couple of workouts.

That doesn't negate what I wrote earlier in the chapter. You never want the exercises to be easy, and you always want to move ahead when you can. But when you return to basic exercises after a long break, they won't be easy. It'll take you a workout or two to restore your endurance, which is exactly why it's important to do just that.

## HOW TO SELECT EXERCISES

Sometimes you'll have two core exercises in each workout, sometimes only one. If there are two core exercises in each workout:

1. Always do one anti-extension (or hip flexion) exercise.
2. The other can be either anti-rotation or anti-lateral flexion.

If there is one core exercise each workout:

1. Always do an anti-extension exercise in one workout, either Workout A or Workout B.
2. Do either an anti-rotation or anti-lateral flexion exercise in the other.

Most readers should simply start with the Level 1 exercise in every category, and move up when you can. It doesn't matter how much experience you have. Just do Level 1 exercises your first workout. If you're an experienced lifter and you blow right past the time limits, you can go up to 60 seconds for planks and 45 seconds per side for side planks.

Still easy? No problem. Do Level 2 exercises the next time you do that workout.

Let's see how this plays out in Basic Training I. Alwyn has you doing two core exercises in each workout, one each from the stabilization and dynamic-stabilization categories.

## WORKOUT A

*Stabilization:* plank (anti-extension, Level 1)

*Dynamic stabilization:* side plank and row (anti-lateral flexion, Level 1)

## WORKOUT B

*Stabilization:* side plank (anti-lateral flexion, Level 1)

*Dynamic stabilization:* front plank and pull-down (anti-extension, Level 1)

With stabilization exercises, as I said, you want to move up a level as soon as you hit the time limit at your current level. You probably won't move forward at the same pace in each category. That's my favorite part of the template system: You move up when you're ready, even if it's in the middle of a program. On the other hand, when you finish one program, you can continue with the same stabilization exercises in the next one, if you're still improving.

For dynamic stabilization, you want to advance when you can't increase the weight, or max out on the reps, or finish your current program. If you do the exercise for an entire program of four to six weeks, you're ready for something else, even if you're still making progress.

So what about anti-rotation, the third type of core exercise? When you get to Basic Training II, do the first anti-rotation option (the tall kneeling static hold, shown on page 181) as your stabilization exercise.

STABILIZATION LEVEL 1

# ✳ Plank (anti-extension)

**BEST FOR:** everyone to start with. This is the ur-stabilization exercise. Just as all politics is local, so does all core stability begin with the basic plank. Some experienced lifters may only use it for one workout, while beginners will work at it for a while to build their endurance.

### GET READY/HOLD

- You'll need either a well-padded floor, or a mat to put under your forearms.
- Get into plank position, which is also called a modified push-up position: You're facedown, with your weight resting on your forearms and toes and your body in a straight line from neck to ankles. Your upper arms are perpendicular to the floor, with your elbows directly beneath your shoulders.
- Hold that position for up to 30 seconds.
- If 30 seconds is easy, you can hold up to 60 seconds, and do a more challenging plank variation the next time you repeat the workout.

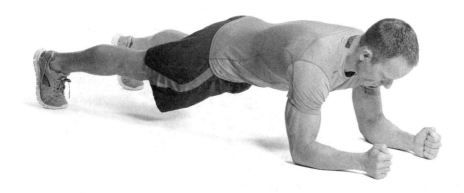

## ✳ Side plank (anti-lateral flexion)

**BEST FOR:** same as the plank: Everyone will start here. Some will move on, while beginners will work at the side plank for a while to build their endurance.

**GET READY/HOLD**

- Lie on your left side with your legs straight and your right leg on top of your left. Position yourself so your weight rests on your left forearm and the outside edge of your left foot. Your left elbow should be directly beneath your shoulder, with your upper arm perpendicular to the floor.
- Lift your hips until your body is in a straight line from neck to ankles. You want your shoulders square and on a plane that's perpendicular to the floor, as if your back was supported by a wall.
- You can place your right hand on your right hip, as shown, or left shoulder.
- Hold that position for up to 30 seconds, then switch sides and repeat.
- If 30 seconds is easy, you can hold up to 45 seconds, and do a more challenging side-plank variation the next time you repeat the workout.

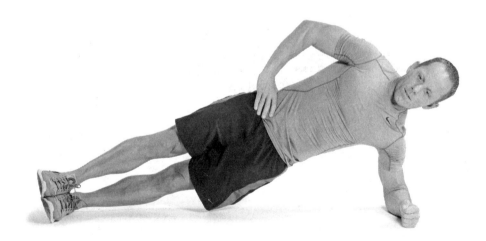

## ✳ Cable tall kneeling static hold (anti-rotation)

**BEST FOR:** This is the exercise you need to master before you move on to the chops in the Dynamic Stabilization category. It looks simple enough, but if you've never done it before, you can't predict how your body will respond to this unusual challenge to your torso muscles. I see lots of people doing a dynamic version of this exercise called a Pallof press, in which you press your hands out from your chest and then pull them back, rather than simply holding with your arms extended. When it's performed incorrectly (which is most of the time, in my experience), it's because the user hasn't mastered the static hold, which is the most important part.

### GET READY
- Attach a D-shaped handle to the cable pulley, and set it to mid-thigh height.
- You can also do this with a band, as long as you can attach it to something sturdy that's about 30 inches above the floor (depending on your height).

### HOLD
- Grab the handle with both hands and kneel sideways to the machine.
- Straighten your torso so your body is on a single plane from ears to knees, with your hips and shoulders square.
- Hold the handle straight out in front of your chest for 30 seconds, then switch sides and repeat.
- The key is keeping your shoulders and hips aligned as your core muscles fatigue. This is the part that most people I see doing the Pallof press can't yet manage.

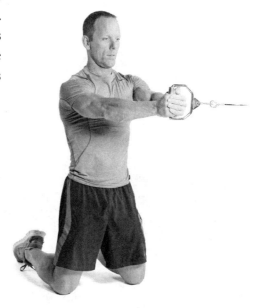

**STABILIZATION LEVEL 2**

## ✳ Plank with reduced base of support (anti-extension)

**BEST FOR:**  Everyone should reach this progression during Basic Training. This is the part of core training in which you go from building pure endurance to improving coordination and fatigue resistance.

**GET READY/HOLD**

- From the basic plank position, you can:
  - Lift one leg.
  - Lift one arm, extending it in front of you.
- You can maintain any of these positions for an entire 30-second set, and then repeat with the opposite limbs elevated. Or you can raise one limb for half the time, then switch for the other half of the set.
- If you reach the maximum time with either the arm or leg raise, there's no need to repeat it in a subsequent workout. Just make sure you've hit maximum time with both options before you move on to the next level.

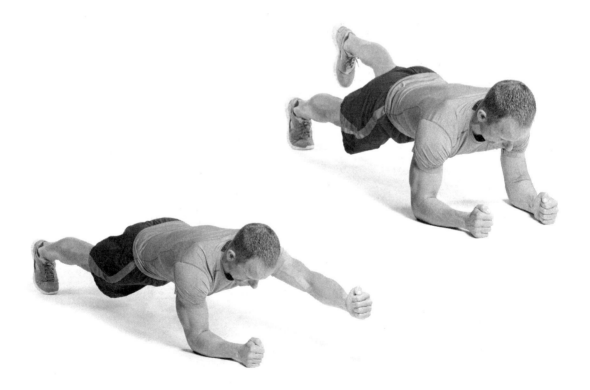

### SUPERCHARGE IT!

You can also run through the same series from the push-up position. These are my two favorite Level 2 stabilization exercises:

- From the push-up position, lift one hand and raise it to your chest. If you can hold for 30 seconds with each hand on your chest (with or without a break in between), you're in pretty good shape.
- From the push-up position, lift one arm and the opposite-side leg. If you can hold each side for 30 seconds, you're far more awesome than I. (With practice, I can do a total of 60 seconds, but only if I switch sides every 15 seconds.)

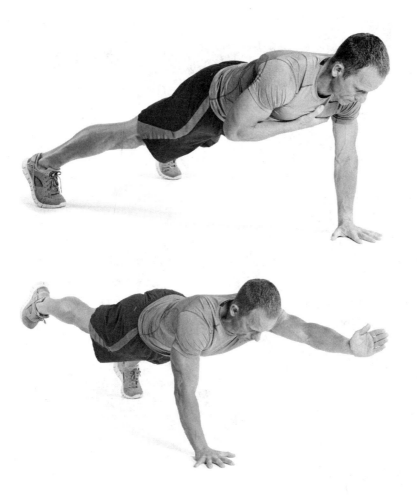

## ✳ Side plank with reduced base of support (anti-lateral flexion)

**BEST FOR:** This is a much tougher progression than the ones in the plank series. You're going to feel it in your abductors, the outer-hip muscles.

### GET READY/HOLD

- Get into the side-plank position and lift your top leg so your legs form a V shape.
- A 30-second hold is probably too ambitious. Shoot for 15 seconds per side per set, but always do at least 2 sets.

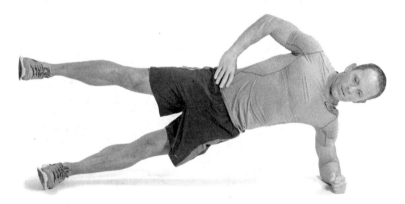

### SUPERCHARGE IT!

The side plank with knee tuck always seems like a good idea, until I'm halfway through a 30-second hold and start questioning my life choices. Lift your bottom leg off the floor, bending your hip and knee so your bottom foot is near your top knee. Your weight will rest on your forearm and the inside edge of your top foot. You're going to feel it on the inside of your top leg, which has the burden of supporting most of your body weight.

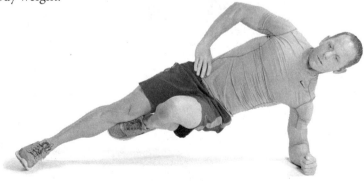

## ✴ Cable half-kneeling static hold (anti-rotation)

**BEST FOR:** a simple progression from the tall kneeling static hold. This is the last pure anti-rotation exercise in the stabilization category. But as you'll see when you try the Level 3, 4, and 5 plank variations, the challenges to your stability, strength, endurance, and balance come from all directions.

**GET READY/HOLD**

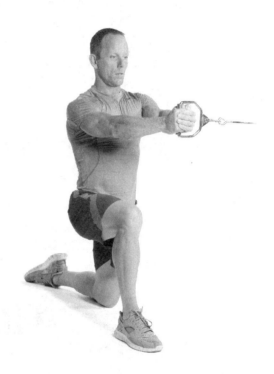

- Set up as described for the Level 1 static hold, with the knee closest to the cable machine on the floor.
- With your torso straight and shoulders square, hold the handle out in front of your chest with straight arms for 30 seconds.
- Switch sides and repeat.

### STABILIZATION LEVEL 3

## ✴ Feet-elevated plank (anti-extension)

This one is just like it sounds: Set your feet on a box or step that's about 6 to 12 inches high. If you're using a higher step or bench, go to the push-up hold. It's a pretty easy progression either way. The real fun begins again at Level 4.

## ✴ Feet-elevated side plank (anti-lateral flexion)

Same as above: Set your feet on a low box or step. For me this is substantially harder than the feet-elevated plank.

### STABILIZATION LEVEL 4

## ✳ Feet-elevated push-up hold with reduced base of support (anti-extension)

This is a fun, challenging progression. I recommend doing all these from the push-up position. Unless you have a very low box or step (6 inches or less), it's going to be hard to maintain a neutral spine from the plank position with your feet elevated and an arm or leg in the air. And there isn't much point in doing a stability exercise, no matter how challenging, while stabilizing the wrong position.

Your options include:

- Raise one leg.
- Raise one arm.
- Raise one leg and the opposite-side arm.

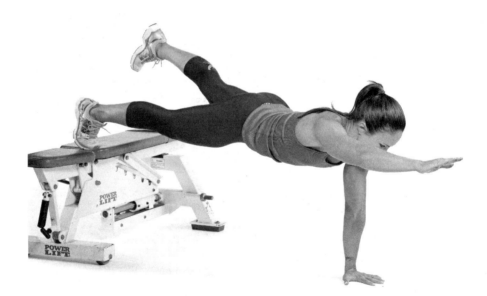

## ✳ Feet-elevated side plank with reduced base of support (anti-lateral flexion)

Yet again, these options are a lot harder, and a lot less fun, than the corresponding options for the plank or push-up hold. I don't recommend doing these with a step or box that's higher than 12 inches.

Your options include:

- Raise your top leg so your legs form a V shape.
- Lift and tuck your bottom leg.

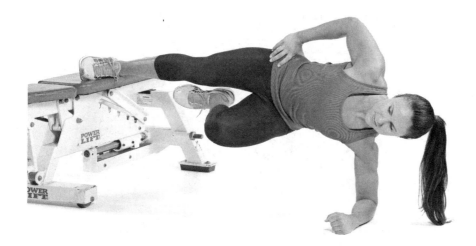

### STABILIZATION LEVEL 5

## ✳ Feet-elevated plank or push-up hold with unstable point of contact (anti-extension)

**BEST FOR:** advanced lifters who want to do exercises that sometimes offer an adrenaline rush along with fitness benefits.

Possibilities include:

- Elevate your feet on a Swiss ball with your hands on the floor.
- Suspend your feet with a TRX or equivalent, hands on floor.
- Elevate your feet on a stable platform (box or bench), and put your hands on or in something unstable:
  - Swiss ball
  - One or two medicine balls
  - Suspension system

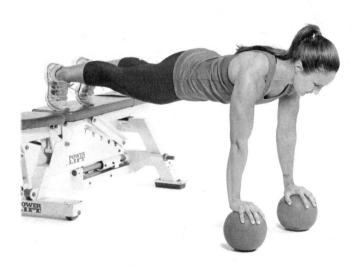

### SUPERCHARGE IT!

Feeling adventurous? Try a push-up hold with (1) feet elevated, (2) hands or feet on an unstable object, and (3) one arm or leg elevated, reducing the point of contact.

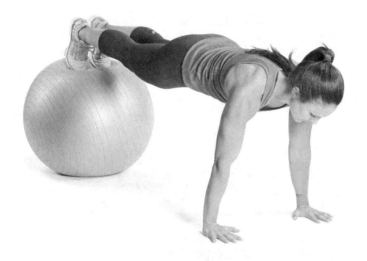

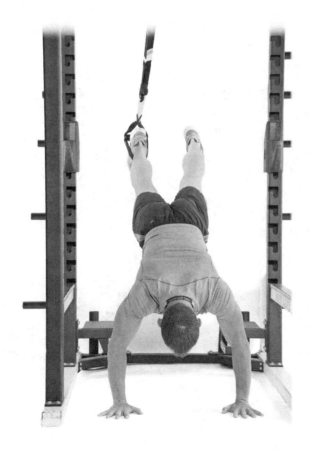

## ✳ Swiss-ball side plank (anti-lateral flexion)

It's pretty awkward to do a side plank with both feet on a Swiss ball, but this version, with the Swiss ball between your feet, is challenging without being stupid-hard to pull off.

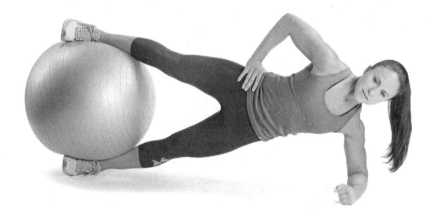

### SUPERCHARGE IT!

I don't know if the suspended side plank is substantially harder, but I'm sure it's more versatile. Whereas there's no way to progress the Swiss-ball side plank, on this one you can:

- Start with both feet suspended.
- Suspend the bottom foot, with the top foot free.
- Suspend the top foot, and tuck the bottom foot against your top leg.

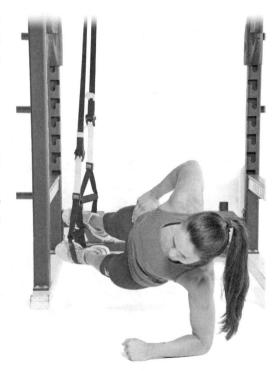

**DYNAMIC STABILIZATION LEVEL 1**

# ✳ Plank and pulldown (anti-extension)

**BEST FOR:** everyone. Enjoyed by: no one. This exercise is an equal-opportunity slice of "you're not as good as you think." I wouldn't do it if Alwyn didn't write it into the programs. Even the models want overtime pay when we make them do it for photos. It's not a difficult exercise. It's just awkward. But if nothing else, it lets you experience just how much your lats contribute to core stability when you're in the plank position. Calling on them to do two things at once—pulling and stabilizing—exposes your weaknesses in both areas. Which is exactly why Alwyn includes it.

**GET READY**

- Attach a D-shaped handle to the low cable pulley. You can also use a band attached to a point a few inches above the floor.
- Set up in the plank position facing the cable machine, feet set wide for extra stability.
- Grab the handle with your right hand, using a neutral grip (your palm facing in, neither underhand nor overhand). You'll probably have to reposition yourself to establish tension in the cable when your arm is fully extended in front of you.

**MOVE**

- Pull the handle until it's just below your shoulder and your upper arm is alongside your torso.
- Keep the rest of your body in the plank position, with a neutral spine and your chest and hips square to the floor.
- Do all your reps, switch sides, and repeat.

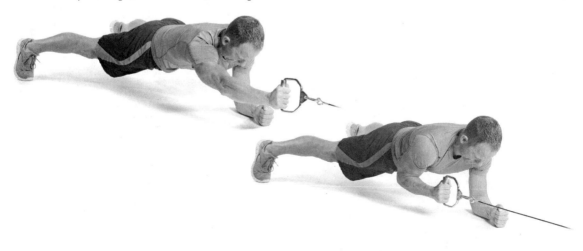

## ✳ Side plank and row (anti-lateral flexion)

**BEST FOR:** everybody, and hated by nobody. It's a pretty simple and easy exercise compared to the plank and pulldown. This time you have your trapezius and rear deltoids helping your lats execute the pull, while your primary stabilizing muscles (obliques, rectus abdominis, spinal erectors, quadratus lumborum) aren't forced to do double duty. Alwyn considers this an anti-rotation exercise as well as one that prevents lateral flexion.

### GET READY

- Attach a D-shaped handle to the low cable pulley (or use a band at a similar attachment point).
- Get into side-plank position facing the cable machine, supporting your weight on your left side.
- Grab the handle with your right hand, palm facing down, and adjust your position so your arm is fully extended toward the machine with tension on the cable.

### MOVE

- Pull the handle to the right side of your rib cage, keeping your body aligned on a plane perpendicular to the floor.
- Do all your reps, switch sides, and repeat.
- Word of warning: Don't get too ambitious with the weights here; the goal isn't to build your lats, it's to maintain a stable position with one limb moving in a different plane.

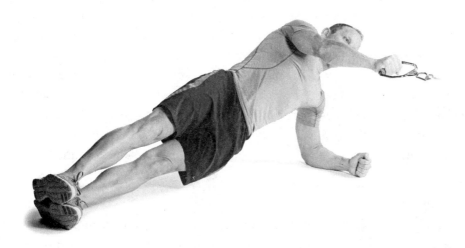

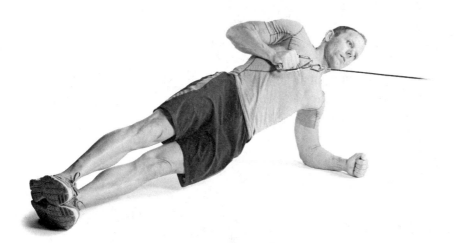

### DYNAMIC STABILIZATION LEVEL 2

## ✳ Push-away (anti-extension)

**BEST FOR:** an introduction to perhaps the most effective and challenging series of core exercises you can attempt. Once you have a base of core strength and endurance, this exercise teaches you to resist spinal extension while your center of gravity moves away from your core. The most often seen version is the rollout, usually done with an ab wheel (a lawnmower wheel with handles) or a barbell. Those rollouts are performed from the knees, which is why Alwyn doesn't include them in the NROL programs. They're incredibly tough exercises, and they'll leave your abs sore for days the first time you try them, but there's no simple progression from the knees to a standing position.

**GET READY**

- Grab a pair of Valslides, furniture sliders, or anything else that will slip across your floor with minimal friction while supporting your weight. (Towels should work on a wood or tile floor, while plastic works best on a carpet.)
- Get into push-up position with one slide in each hand.

**MOVE**

- Slide your right arm as far forward as you can, keeping your arm straight and your core in a stable, neutral position. If you feel anything move in your lower back, shorten your range of motion.
- Pull it back, then slide your left arm forward.
- Alternate until you finish the set. If the workout calls for 10 reps, do that many with each arm.

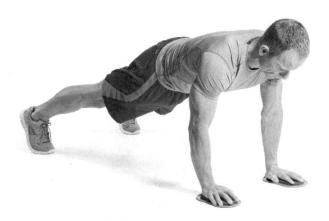

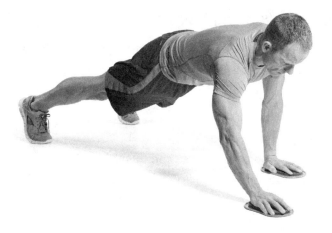

## SUPERCHARGE IT!

If you're an advanced lifter in both core and upper-body strength, you can try the push-away with bent arms. From the same starting position, push your right arm as far forward as you can, bending your left elbow and lowering your chest toward the floor, as if you were doing a push-up. Pull your arm back, and repeat with your left arm. Each of those—left and right—counts as a repetition, so a set of 10 would mean 5 reps with each arm. Use this one cautiously; it's more of a Level 4 or 5 variation than Level 2.

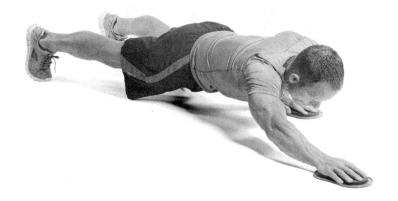

## ✳ Mountain climber (hip flexion)

**BEST FOR:**  Here we introduce a new category of core exercise (for an explanation, see the sidebar). You can use hip-flexion exercises along with or instead of anti-extension exercises.

### GET READY/MOVE

- Get into push-up position on the floor.
- Lift one knee up toward your chest, and then back down.
- As soon as that foot touches the floor, raise the opposite knee.

### Slightly Easier Entry-Level Version

Some of you will do better with your hands elevated on a bench, instead of on the floor, especially if you have short arms and/or long legs.

### SUPERCHARGE IT!

You can also do this with your feet on Valslides or the equivalent. I like it because I can work faster and reach a deeper level of fatigue.

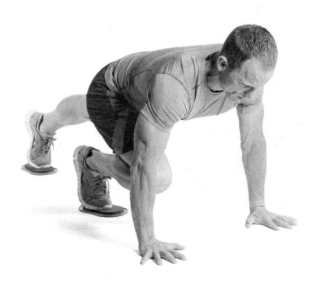

## Hip Ops

Hip flexion is a simple and vital human movement; you use it every time you lift your legs to walk, run, or climb. But there was a time when hip flexion was something you didn't do in polite company. Trainers would walk up to you in the gym, unprompted, to tell you that the sit-up you were doing involved hip flexion, which would lead to a back injury. That's because one of your biggest hip-flexing muscles, the psoas major, originates on the bones of your lower back. From there it crosses the front of your pelvis and attaches to your femur (the hip bone). The idea was that when you shorten the psoas during a hip-flexing exercise, it would pull your lower back out of its natural arch. Thus, hip flexion = back extension, something we want to avoid. That's why we do so many anti-extension exercises.

Unfortunately, those trainers misunderstood the mechanism. The sit-up they warned us against produces lumbar flexion, which *flattens* the lower back. That presents its own problems, as you already know, and explains why Alwyn no longer uses sit-ups, crunches, or leg raises in his programs. High activity from the hip flexors increases spinal compression, which is still a problem. It's just different from what the trainers feared.

But just because hip flexion in those exercises is a bad idea for most of us, that doesn't mean it's not important in general. In *Anatomy Trains*, Thomas Myers shows that the hip flexors share connective tissues with inner-thigh muscles below them and the respiratory muscles above. All those muscles get shorter and weaker with extended hours sitting at our desks or behind the wheel when we drive.

Alwyn's program has lots of exercises that stretch them; anytime you do a lunge, whether it's for mobility or strength, you're stretching the hip flexors. But when do you strengthen them? That's where the hip-flexion exercises come in during core training. You perform them with your back in its natural arch, which avoids putting excess loads on the spine. You also do most of them one leg at a time, which allows the supporting muscles of the lower back to work more effectively. Whereas two legs easily and powerfully pull the lower back out of the neutral zone, it's much harder to do that with one leg. When you do use two legs, you'll do so in a facedown position, with gravity helping you resist potentially risky lumbar flexion.

### DYNAMIC STABILIZATION LEVEL 3

## ✳ Swiss-ball rollout (anti-extension)

**BEST FOR:** a great challenge not just to your core stability, but to your rectus abdominis, which has to lengthen while helping to keep your back in the neutral zone.

**GET READY**

- Set up in plank position with your forearms on the Swiss ball and your toes on the floor.
- Set your body in two straight lines—neck to hips, and hips to ankles—with your body slightly flexed at the hips and your back in the neutral position.

**MOVE**

- Roll the ball forward, straightening your arms and lowering your torso as far as you can while keeping your back in its natural arch.
- Pull back to the starting position.

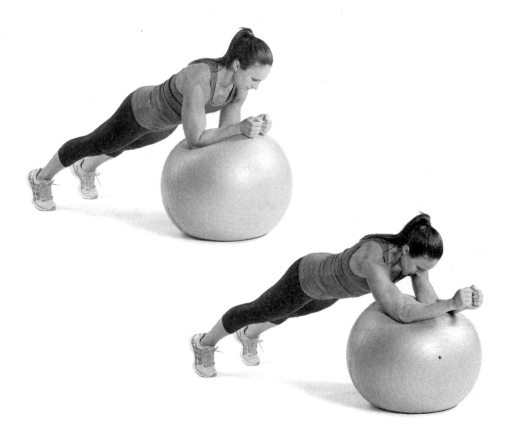

## ✳ Cable tall kneeling chop (anti-rotation)

**BEST FOR:** This exercise is increasingly common, but good form is rare. Inexperienced lifters try to move fast without first establishing a stable base. Experienced lifters often use too much weight, and turn it into a kind of twisting crunch from the knees.

**GET READY**

- Attach a rope handle to the high cable pulley. Pull the rope through its metal attachment ring as far as you can, giving you about 24 inches of rope to grasp.
- Grab the rope with an overhand grip, one hand at each end.
- Kneel sideways to the machine, and straighten your torso so your body is on a single plane from ears to knees, with your shoulders and hips square.

**MOVE**

- Pull the rope down and across your torso. The hand closest to the machine should end up in front of your outside hip. Keep your arms straight and your midsection and hips stationary, moving only your arms and shoulders.
- Do all your reps, switch sides, and repeat.

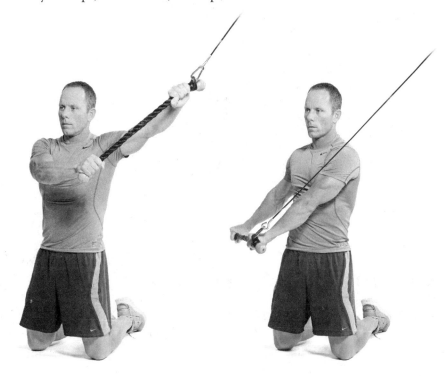

## ✳ Swiss-ball mountain climber (hip flexion)

**BEST FOR:** For some readers, this may be easier than the mountain climber with your hands on the floor, even though you're adding an instability challenge that should make it harder. But with your torso at a steeper angle, it may take less effort to keep your lower back in the neutral zone.

**GET READY**

- Place your hands on a Swiss ball, roughly shoulder-width apart.
- Set up as you would for a push-up hold, with your body in a straight line from neck to ankles.

**MOVE**

- Raise your right leg off the floor and bring your knee up toward your chest.
- Lower it, then repeat with your left.
- Continue alternating until you do all your reps with both legs.

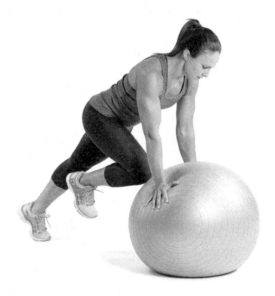

**DYNAMIC STABILIZATION LEVEL 4**

## ✳ Suspended fallout (anti-extension)

**BEST FOR:** a challenging progression from the Swiss-ball rollout, since the range of motion is much greater. The longer the range of motion, the bigger the potential benefit. But with more benefit comes more risk. You have to work at this one a while to get a feel not just for the exercise itself, but for the point at which your back starts to shift out of its neutral zone. That's your limit, and it takes time and effort to figure out where it is, and learn how to stop yourself right before you reach it.

### GET READY
- It will take a few tries to figure out how low to set the handles on the suspension trainer. Higher is better to start. Lower is harder.
- Grab the handles and set up in push-up position, with your body straight from neck to hips and from hips to ankles, with a slight hinge in the middle.

### MOVE
- Fall forward slowly and carefully, lifting your arms out in front of you as your body moves down toward the floor. Keep the exact same hinge in your hips.
- Stop when you reach the deepest point possible while keeping your spine in the neutral position.
- Pull back to the starting position.

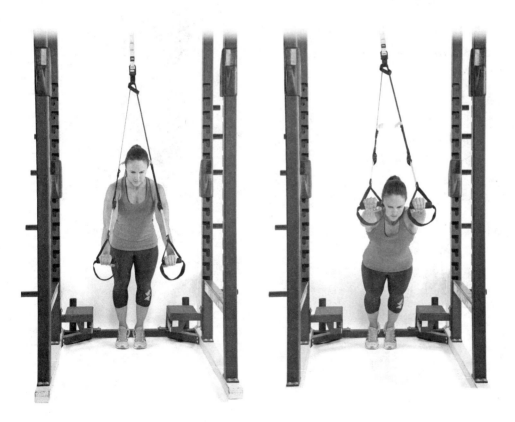

## ✳ Cable half-kneeling chop (anti-rotation)

**BEST FOR:** This is a simple progression from the tall kneeling chop. The only difference is that you've narrowed your base of support.

### GET READY/MOVE

- Set up as you did for the tall kneeling chop, only with your weight resting on one foot (the one closest to the machine) and one knee (the one farthest from it). Lift your torso to make yourself as tall as possible.
- Pull the rope down and across your torso until the hand closest to the machine is in front of your outside hip.
- Do all your reps, switch sides, and repeat.

## ✳ Swiss-ball jackknife (hip flexion)

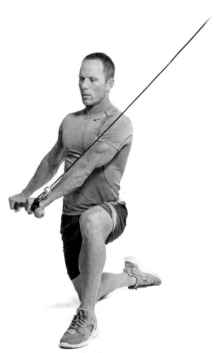

**BEST FOR:** a challenging way to do hip flexion, using both legs and an unstable point of contact.

### GET READY

- Set up in push-up position with your hands on the floor and your shins and the tops of your feet on a Swiss ball.
- Set your body in a straight line from ears to ankles.

### MOVE

- Pull your knees forward as far as you can, while keeping your back flat.
- Push the ball back to the starting position.

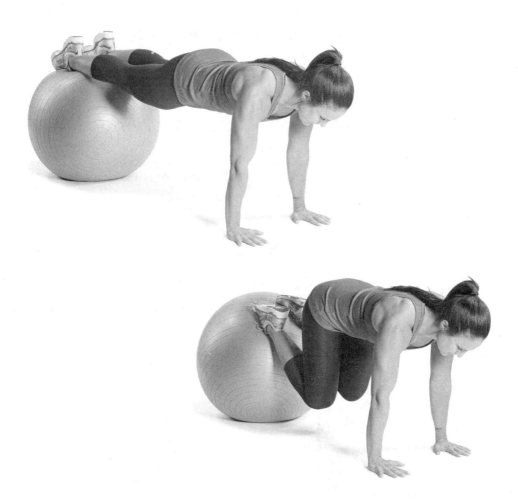

## DYNAMIC/INTEGRATED STABILIZATION LEVEL 5

"Dynamic" and "integrated" are technically separate categories of core training, but here we present the latter as a progression from the former. The reality is that advanced lifters are doing a lot of integrated-stabilization exercises throughout Alwyn's programs. Exercises like the crossover step-ups on page 166, the carries in Chapter 16, and even some of the push-up variations in Chapter 10 require you to stabilize your core during complex movements with a load that's unbalanced in one way or another.

## ✳ Suspended jackknife and push-up (hip flexion)

**BEST FOR:**  Adding a push-up increases the core challenge. First you're trying to avoid rounding your back while doing hip flexion (the jackknife). Then you're resisting back extension during the push-up. If you don't have a suspension trainer, you can add a push-up to the Swiss-ball jackknife and get the same effect.

**GET READY**
- Set the handles of the core trainer about 12 inches from the floor.
- Put your feet in the loops, and set up in push-up position.

**MOVE**
- Pull your knees forward as far as you can while keeping your back in the neutral position.
- As they go back toward the starting position, do a push-up.
- It'll take a couple of tries, but you should be able to establish a good rhythm soon enough.

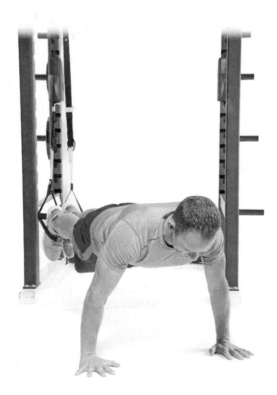

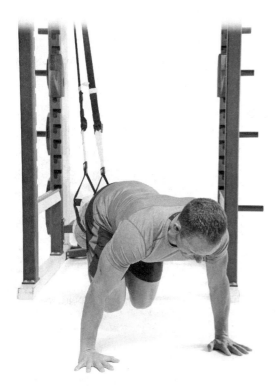

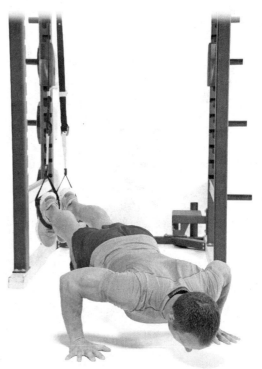

## ✳ Cable chop and reverse lunge (anti-rotation)

**BEST FOR:** putting two now-familiar exercises together to create a multidirectional core challenge.

### GET READY

- Affix the rope attachment to the high cable pulley, as described earlier.
- Stand sideways to the machine, holding the rope between your shoulders and the cable machine, with your feet hip-width apart and your hips and shoulders square.

### MOVE

- Step back in a reverse lunge with the leg farthest from the machine.
- At the same time, pull the rope down and across your torso so the hand closest to the machine ends up in front of your outside hip.
- Return to the starting position, do all your reps, switch sides, and repeat.

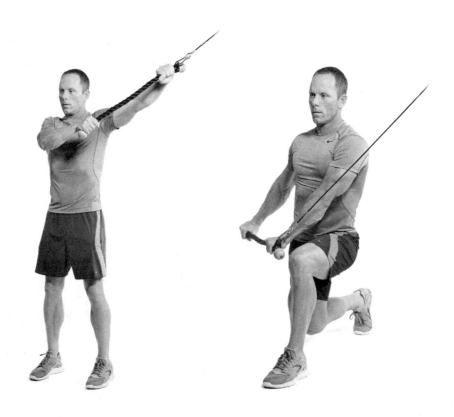

# ✳ Turkish get-up (anti-lateral flexion)

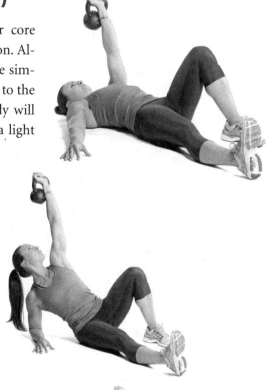

**BEST FOR:** an exercise that challenges your core strength along with your stability and coordination. Although the instructions are complex, the goals are simple: get up from the floor and then get back down to the floor while holding a weight overhead. Your body will figure out the details on its own. Just start with a light weight as you learn the exercise. When you get good at it, and start using heavier weights, you'll want to do lower reps than the workouts prescribe. Five reps per side per set are plenty with challenging weights, and three or four per side may be better.

## GET READY

- Grab a kettlebell (although a dumbbell will work) with your left hand and lie flat on your back on the floor.
- Hold the weight with a straight arm (elbow locked) over your chest.
- Your left knee is bent, with your left foot flat on the floor, toes turned out slightly.
- Your right leg is straight and flat on the floor.
- Your right arm is straight, flat on the floor, palm down, and angled out about 45 degrees from your torso.
- Your eyes are focused on the weight, where they'll stay throughout the movement.

## MOVE

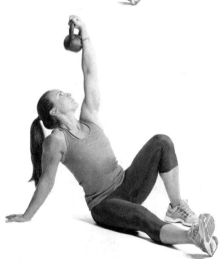

- Push down hard with your left heel as you raise your torso. This is the closest we get to a crunch in the program.
- At the same time, bend your right arm and slide it up so you're supporting your weight first on your right elbow and forearm, then on the palm of your right hand as you straighten your arm. Your right hand

will be slightly behind your torso at this point.

- Push down with your left heel and right hand, lifting your torso and hips off the floor into what some trainers call the "high bridge" position. Hold this position for a second or two.
- Slide your right leg under your body, then rest your right knee on the floor, just beneath your hips.
- Pick your right hand up off the floor and raise your torso. Your weight is now supported by your left foot and right knee.
- Stand up.
- Reverse the steps to get back down to the floor.
- Do all your reps, and repeat on the other side.

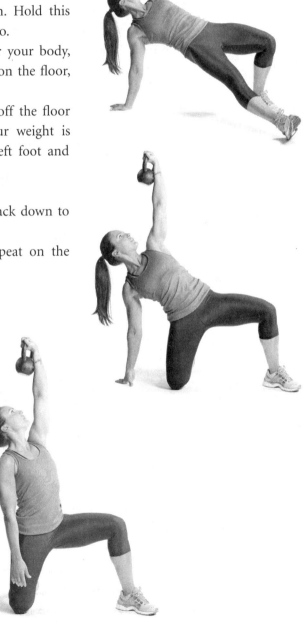

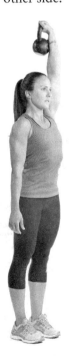

# Combination and Power Exercises

You'll use these exercises in Basic Training. In the first two programs, you'll do one of each per program (a power exercise in the A workout and a combination exercise in B, for example). In Basic Training III you'll do both in A and B, and in Basic Training IV you'll do a combination exercise in both workouts, but no power.

The differences between the two categories are easy to define. A combination exercise involves two distinct movement patterns—a squat with a shoulder press, for example, or a Romanian deadlift with a bent-over row. A power exercise is typically an explosive version of a standard exercise, like a jump squat or push-up in which your hands come all the way off the floor.

But as you gain confidence in the weight room, I think you'll see more similarities than differences. For example, when I do a squat with a shoulder press, I'm not doing either part of the exercise slowly. On the way up I use the momentum of the squat to help me press the weights, and on the way down the momentum allows me to use my muscles' stretch reflex to reverse directions and rise quickly and powerfully out of the squat position. I'm not trying to do the exercises with heavy weights. I'm using moderate weights and relatively fast reps.

When you do power exercises, your goal is similar: use moderate weights and the fastest repetitions possible. Sometimes you want to stop between reps to reset your body, but other times you're doing the exercise rhythmically *and* fast.

That's where the benefits spill over and become indistinguishable. All the exercises in both categories require a higher level of focus, and help you develop better coordination. They're harder to do, which means you'll need a bit more time to catch your breath between sets. You'll do them faster than typical exercises, either by design with power training or necessity with the combo moves.

One more common trait: You'll either love them or hate them with equivalent passion. It's hard to remain neutral with exercises that make you do something you aren't used to doing.

### COMBINATION LEVEL 1

## ✳ Reverse lunge and shoulder press

**BEST FOR:** Most readers can start with this one for Basic Training I. The one exception will be advanced lifters who don't want to do two lunge variations in the same workout. (Basic Training I, Workout B, includes lunges.) Remember that you're doing all the prescribed reps with both legs, which means twice that many shoulder presses. Choose your weights appropriately.

**GET READY/MOVE**
- Grab a pair of dumbbells and hold them at your shoulders, with your palms turned toward each other.
- Stand with your feet hip-width apart.
- Take a long step back with your right leg, pressing the weights overhead as you drop into a lunge position, with your right knee nearly touching the floor.
- Step back to the starting position as you lower the weights to your shoulders.
- Do all your reps, switch legs, and repeat.

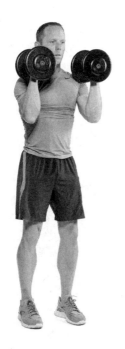

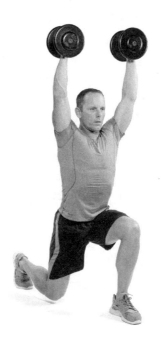

## SUPERCHARGE IT!

Experienced readers can try the exercise pressing one weight at a time, using a dumbbell or kettlebell. Hold the weight in your right hand when you step back with your right leg, and vice versa. Since you're pressing with one arm at a time, you should be able to use a heavier weight.

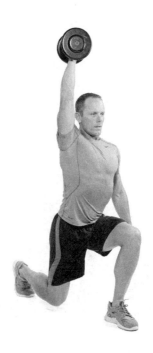

## COMBINATION LEVEL 2

## ✳ Romanian deadlift and row

**BEST FOR:** This is a good choice for anyone, with the possible exception of those who have lower-back issues. For the stronger and more experienced lifters, it's a great choice for those workouts when you need to do a combination exercise in addition to a squat or a lunge. The deadlift part won't be excessively taxing, since you're using a weight that's more appropriate for the rows. So it's like having an extra upper-body exercise, but with more metabolic benefits.

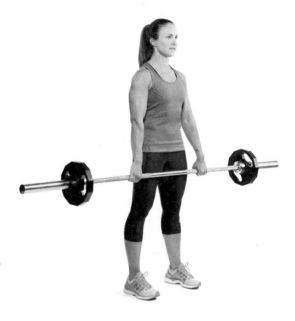

### GET READY/MOVE

- Grab the barbell overhand, your hands just outside shoulder width. Stand holding it at arm's length against your front thighs, with your feet about shoulder-width apart.
- Push your hips back and lower the bar until it's just below your knees and your torso is parallel to the floor, more or less. Your knees will bend slightly.
- Pull the bar straight up to your lower abdomen while keeping your torso in the same position.

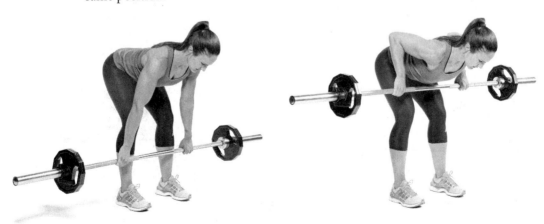

- Lower the bar to arm's length.
- Push your hips forward and return to the starting position. That's one rep.

### COMBINATION LEVEL 3

## ✳ Squat and press

**BEST FOR:**  This is my favorite combination exercise. The movement feels natural, and I can typically use decent weights. But it's one of the most taxing as well. One word of caution: I would avoid using this on days you do squats as a strength exercise, especially if you (like me) have knee issues.

#### GET READY/MOVE

- Grab a pair of dumbbells and hold them at your shoulders, with your palms turned toward each other.
- Stand with your feet shoulder-width apart, toes pointed forward.
- Push your hips back and descend into a squat.
- As you return to the starting position, press the weights straight up over your shoulders. Lower them to the starting position, and immediately drop into a squat to begin the next repetition.

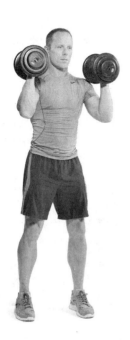
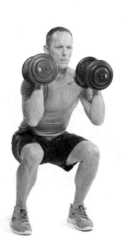
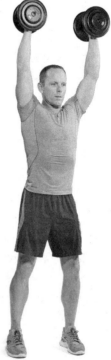

## SUPERCHARGE IT?

The side lunge and press isn't for me, but someone with good knees and out-standing hip mobility could use it to great effect: Set up as you would for the squat and press, take a long step to the side, and drop into a side lunge while pressing the weights overhead. Push back to the starting position and repeat to the other side. Do the prescribed reps to both sides. You get a stability challenge that starts with your shoulders and goes all the way down to your feet and ankles.

### COMBINATION LEVEL 4

## ✳ Push-up and one-arm row

**BEST FOR:** This is a great core exercise, and an outstanding sweat-inducer when your goal is fat loss. But it will frustrate the snot out of anyone who treats it as a muscle-builder. Reasonably strong adults will quickly discover how hard it is to row even 10 pounds for the prescribed reps. I like to use it when I need a break from lower-body training. There's no stress on your knees (as there could be with squats and lunges) or lower back (which could happen with the deadlift and bent-over rows), and the work your upper-body muscles do shouldn't affect your performance else-where in the workout. Just be prepared for a very tough core challenge, and keep a fresh gym towel handy to mop up the floor when you're finished.

**GET READY/MOVE**

- Grab a pair of light dumbbells. (I recommend subtracting at least 25 percent from whatever you *think* you can use the first time you try it.) Hex dumbbells probably work best. Round dumbbells add a bit to the stability challenge, but that's the last thing you need on this one.
- Set up in push-up position with the dumbbells in your hands and your palms facing each other. You probably want your hands less than shoulder-width apart. The closer they are to each other, the easier it will be to execute the row.
- For the same reason, you probably want to start with your feet more than shoulder-width apart.
- Most of us will do this with a slight hinge in our hips, even if we're trying to keep our body in a straight line from neck to ankles. There's no problem with the hinge; just keep your back in the same position throughout the set.

## MOVE

- Lower your chest to the floor, and as you push back up, row the weight in your right hand to the side of your torso.
- Lower the weight to the floor, and execute the next push-up, this time rowing with your left arm. (You can also do this with one arm at a time, which should allow you to use a heavier weight.)
- Continue alternating until you do all the reps with both arms. Keep in mind that this means you'll do twice as many push-ups as the workout specifies.

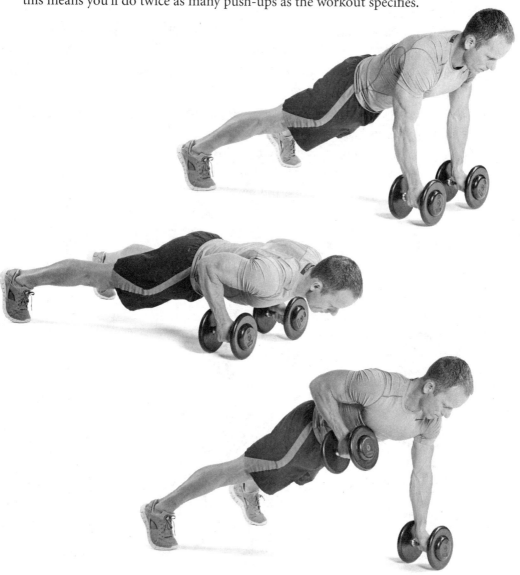

### COMBINATION LEVEL 5

## ✳ Offset squat and one-arm shoulder press

**BEST FOR:** This is an all-around-solid exercise for experienced readers. The off-set load gives you a core challenge. You should be able to use a relatively heavy weight for the press. And because you're doing equal reps on both sides, you end up doing a lot of squats, which increases the metabolic cost.

### GET READY/MOVE

- Grab a kettlebell and hold it in one arm in the rack position (holding the handle near your chin, with the bell resting on the outside of your arm). You can also use a single dumbbell, holding it at your shoulder, with your palm toward the midline of your body.
- Set your feet shoulder-width apart, toes pointed forward or turned out slightly.
- Push your hips back and descend into a squat.
- As you rise back up, press the weight overhead.
- Lower the weight as you descend into the next squat.
- Do all your reps, switch sides, and repeat.

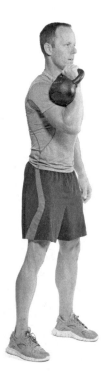
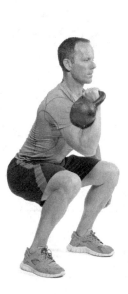
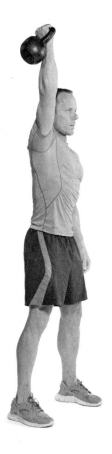

POWER LEVEL 1

### ✳ **Box jump**

**BEST FOR:** everybody. I have to think that anyone who's medically cleared to lift can find a way to do this exercise to beneficial effect, at least until you run out of boxes to jump up to. (I've seen guys put boxes on top of each other and then jump to the top of the stack. It's impressive, but also looks like a skull fracture waiting to happen. Even if I had stones big enough to attempt it, they'd act like an anchor to prevent me from jumping that high.)

**GET READY/MOVE**

- Stand in front of a box or step sturdy enough to support your weight on landing.
- With your feet set shoulder-width apart, bend at the hips and knees as you swing your arms back, then throw your arms forward and jump up onto the box.
- Land with "soft" knees to cushion your landing.
- Step off the box and repeat.
- Advance to a higher box when you can do all the reps with good form. Move up to Level 2 when you run out of higher boxes.

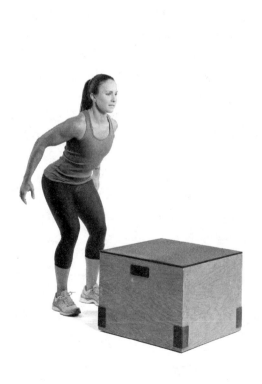
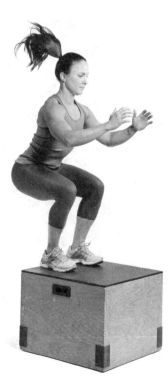

## POWER LEVEL 2

### ✳ Jump squat

**BEST FOR:** On the one hand, it's a straightforward progression from the box jump. On the other, it's the best exercise we have for advanced athletes to improve vertical jump and sprint performance. That comes from Robert Newton, PhD, a professor of sports science at Edith Cowan University in Australia and probably the world's most prolific researcher of power training and development. I e-mailed Dr. Newton to ask about another exercise, the power clean, shown in Chapter 16. I expected him to say it's the best power exercise for athletes. But to my surprise, he told me "the loaded jump squat is superior to about everything else. Time and again our research team and others have proven that even in highly trained individuals, jumping with additional load beyond body weight is highly effective." That's why everyone should use the jump squat for at least one program, and athletes should probably use it for multiple programs.

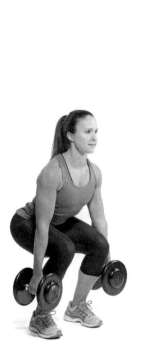
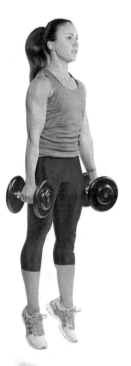

**GET READY/MOVE**

- If you're new to lifting, or just new to this exercise, you should start with just your body weight. Hold your hands behind your head in the prisoner grip.
- More advanced lifters can hold dumbbells at their sides. Alwyn uses a weighted vest with his clients at Results Fitness. If you have one, feel free to use it.
- Set your feet shoulder-width apart with your toes pointed forward.
- Push your hips back until your knees are bent about 90 degrees, and jump.
- Land with soft knees and immediately descend into the next squat.

## POWER LEVEL 3

### ✳ Option 1: Kettlebell swing

**BEST FOR:** I think it works best in Basic Training III, when you're doing a power exercise in each workout. (You can also use it as a metabolic finisher in other programs, if you really like the exercise.) It's a pure hip-extension exercise, meaning there's really nothing else to it. The weight isn't hard to move; you aren't even working against gravity for most of its trajectory. The benefit comes from mastering the hip thrust, which should carry over to other exercises in the hinge category.

**GET READY/MOVE**

- Grab a kettlebell and hold it with both hands in front of your torso, with your arms straight.
- Set your feet about one and a half times shoulder-width apart, your toes angled out.
- Push your hips back, lowering your torso toward the floor as the kettlebell swings back behind you.
- Snap your hips forward as you come back up, propelling the kettlebell up and out in front of your chest. Don't raise it with your shoulders; the height of its trajectory should be determined by the power of your hip thrust.
- Let the kettlebell swing back between your legs as you push your hips back for the next repetition.
- If you don't have a heavy enough kettlebell for the two-arm swing, you can do one-arm swings, using the same technique. Do all the reps with each arm.

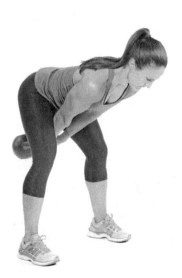
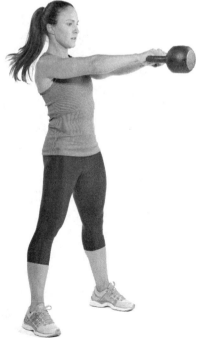

## ✳ Option 2 Explosive push-up

**BEST FOR:** This one is complicated. The push-up is a great exercise, but the explosive push-up, with your hands coming all the way off the floor, may not be a great *power* exercise. The landing can be jarring to your shoulders and especially tough on your wrists. A 2011 study in the *Journal of Strength and Conditioning Research* noted that upper-body muscles and joints don't have the same tolerance for high-impact exercises as the lower body. It compared three types of explosive push-ups, and found that while muscle activation was higher in the one shown here, with your hands rising off the floor, the impact of landing could negate that benefit for many. As an alternative, the researchers showed that doing normal push-ups with maximum speed on the way up and the way down offers similar muscle activation along with higher and faster overall force development. Put another way, you generate more power, and generate it slightly faster, when your hands stay on the floor.

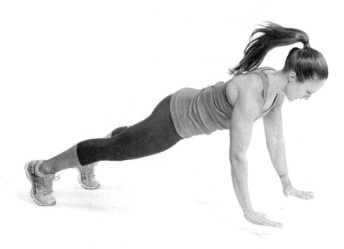

**GET READY/MOVE**

- Set up in push-up position, with your hands on a well-padded surface.
- Bend your elbows and drop toward the floor, but quickly reverse the movement just before impact.
- Push up as hard as you can, with your hands rising off the floor when your arms are straight.
- Land and immediately descend for the next push-up.

POWER LEVEL 4

## ✳ Jump shrug

**BEST FOR:** This is the first power exercise to combine upper- and lower-body action (remember that your arms are just along for the ride in the kettlebell swing), and as such it's both a good exercise on its own and a gateway drug to the more complex Olympic lifts we show in the next chapter. It also works the upper trapezius in a shrugging action, which would seemingly contradict the message of Chapter 11. But we aren't using it to make the upper traps all big and veiny. (Although they will probably be sore for a few days after your first bout of jump shrugs.) The goal is to learn to use that movement to generate force, propelling a weight upward. You'll take the next step—pulling a weight overhead—in Level 5.

**GET READY/ MOVE**

- Grab a barbell with an overhand, shoulder-width grip, and hold it at arm's length in front of you.
- Stand with your feet just a bit less than shoulder-width apart, toes pointed forward.
- Push your hips back and lower the bar until it's just above your knees, which will bend slightly.
- Now you're going to jump by generating power at three joints simultaneously to pull the bar straight up your toward your waistline:
  - Thrust your hips forward
  - Straighten your knees
  - Push up on your toes
- As your feet come off the floor, shrug your shoulders as hard as you can, but keep your arms straight.
- Relax, reset your feet, and start the next rep.

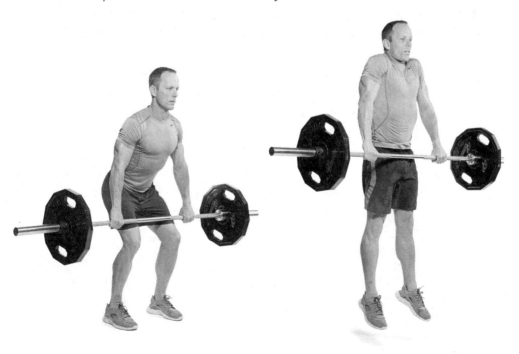

POWER LEVEL 5

## ✳ Dumbbell single-arm snatch

**BEST FOR:** advanced lifters who like the liberating feeling of throwing something heavy overhead (but not letting go). It's sort of like the Turkish get-up shown in Chapter 14, in that the instructions are complex, but the exercise itself is one that your body can learn how to execute without a lot of technical instruction. Moreover, it's a safe exercise for those who've invested some time in the weight room and have the calluses to show for it. You have to be confident that you won't hit yourself or anyone else with the weight (or inadvertently let go of it mid-flight), but how hard is that? Clear some space before you lift, remember to move your head out of the way, and you're all set.

### GET READY/MOVE

- Grab a dumbbell with your right hand and stand with your feet shoulder-width apart, toes pointed forward.
- Push your hips back and bend your knees, with the dumbbell hanging straight down from your shoulder between your legs, palm facing behind you.
- Jump, powering the movement with your hips, knees, and ankles, and coming all the way up on your toes, or even off the floor slightly.
- Shrug your shoulder as you come up, which will pull the weight up the front of your torso. Allow your arm to bend so the weight will be near your chin at the top of the jump.
- At the top, flip your wrist around so your palm faces forward.
- As your body comes down, straighten your arm so the weight ends up overhead. Your knees and hips will be bent slightly, as they would be when you land after a jump. Keep in mind that you aren't lifting with your arm. You straighten your arm as you duck under the weight.
- Catch your balance and stand up straight to complete the repetition, then drop the weight back to the starting position and begin the next snatch.
- Do all the reps, then repeat the set with your other arm.

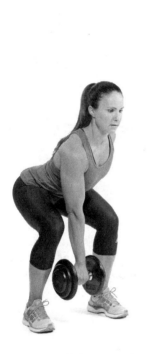
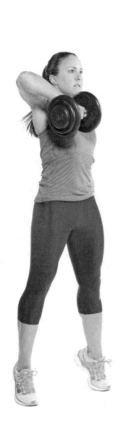
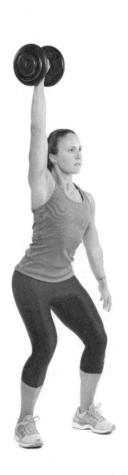

# 16

# Metabolic Training

AT THE END OF EACH *Supercharged* workout you'll do some type of metabolic training. The specifics differ from program to program, but you'll find three major approaches:

## INTERVALS

In traditional interval training, you would do an endurance activity—running, cycling, swimming—for a specific amount of time, and then rest for some multiple of that time. You might run for 60 seconds and rest for 120 seconds. Or it might be 30 seconds of movement followed by 60 seconds of rest. A more advanced athlete might do 30 seconds of work followed by 30 seconds of rest.

What I have just described is exactly what you'll do at the end of every workout in Basic Training I, II, and III. (Alwyn uses a differently fiendish approach in Basic Training IV; you'll see what I mean in Chapter 19.) *How* you do it, though, is completely up to you. You can run if you want. If you can go outdoors or have access to an indoor track, it's probably a good choice for the 60-second intervals in Basic Training I. But you're not limited to that, or to anything else.

Some possibilities:

- Jumping rope
- Kettlebell swings
- Jumping jacks
- Calisthenics (combination of push-ups and body-weight squats, for example)
- Shadow boxing
- Loaded carries (you'll see examples later in the chapter)
- Walking lunges (a type of loaded carry)
- Battling ropes (a total-body conditioning system invented by strongman John Brookfield, in which you create waves with long, thick, heavy ropes)
- Sledgehammer strikes on a tire
- Miscellaneous locomotion exercises (explained in a moment)

You can even use your gym's cardio machines. The rowing machine could be a great choice for the longer intervals. Another would be an Airdyne stationary bike (it's the one with the front wheel that looks like a giant fan). Alwyn wouldn't use a treadmill, elliptical, stairclimber, or standard stationary bike with his clients, but that doesn't mean you can't or shouldn't use one of those machines if they're the best available option and you like using them.

What matters most is that you do the intervals. It's not that you're going to get a huge weight-loss stimulus from a few minutes' worth of exercise at the end of the workout. The significance comes from the fact that you're doing that exercise in a deep state of fatigue. It's an additive benefit, increasing the metabolic cost of the workout (and thus the amount of time your metabolism will remain elevated following the workout as you recover) while improving your conditioning level over time.

## COMPLEXES

These are strength-exercise combinations that you do at the end of the workouts in Hypertrophy I, II, and III. For example, you might do a three-exercise complex with a barbell in which you don't put the weight down until you've done all the reps of all three exercises. But you can use anything you have available. You could do one exercise with dumbbells, the next with a band, and the third with your body weight. As long as you follow the protocol—do all the reps fast, and don't rest between exercises— you'll get the benefits.

Alwyn prescribes sets, reps, and rest periods, and we give you some examples of complexes later in this chapter. You get to choose the exercises and equipment. You probably want to use two different complexes in each Hypertrophy program, one each for workouts A and B.

Whatever you choose, Alwyn recommends that you stick with it for the entire program. That way you can keep track of your results, increasing both the volume and the amount of weight.

Speaking of volume, this is as good a time as any to explain something that applies to all metabolic training, in all programs. The designated sets and reps are a target that not all of us can or will hit. Me, I'm absolutely fried after one of Alwyn's strength workouts. I don't hold anything back, and after 45 to 50 minutes I'm lucky to get through *half* the metabolic training.

It's the effort that matters, not the result. If you've done all you can, that's exactly when Alwyn would stop your workout, if he were training you one-on-one. Stop training, start recovering, and try to build on what you accomplished in your next workout.

## FREE ZONE

Alwyn used to call these "finishers," a word that means something specific to gym rats that's different from his intention. In bodybuilding, a "finisher" is an exercise that puts a cherry on top of whatever the goal of the workout happened to be. That's not what Alwyn has in mind for the final minutes of Strength & Power I, II, and III. You can do anything you want at the end of those workouts, as long as you do it in this specific way:

1. Pick any two strength exercises, which you'll alternate.
2. Do 8 to 10 reps per exercise.
3. Do as many sets of each exercise as you can in 5 minutes.
4. Try to do more the next time you do that workout.

You have infinite possibilities. Alwyn says that the guys at Results Fitness will typically want to do arm exercises, one each for biceps and triceps. Women will usually choose lower-body exercises. You can pick any two exercises in this book, or any other book. It's up to you to decide if the exercises make sense in the context of your own program.

Strength & Power I has two workouts, each of which you'll do six times before moving on. S&P II and III have four—A, B, C, and D—and you'll do each three times. Either way, it's a total of twelve workouts per program. You probably want to keep it simple and come up with two different Free Zone exercise pairs for each program. If you don't like them you can change them up whenever you want, even if it's in the middle of a program. Or, if you love them, you can continue with the same ones for multiple programs.

It seems like a good idea to do a pair of exercises at least two or three times so you can chart your progress. But it wouldn't be a Free Zone if that were a rule. When I get to that part of the workout, I feel like I'm done with charting. I rotate two or three pairs of exercises, and hope I can remember from one time to the next how much weight I used and how many sets I finished. Honestly, I don't care all that much. The point isn't to create a quantifiable training effect. It's to create a feeling, or to combat a feeling.

So if I'm feeling small, I'll do a pair of upper-body exercises that make me feel, for lack of a better word, *swole* (a running joke with a couple of the trainers at my gym). If I'm feeling flabby, I'll do something a little more metabolically demanding. I might choose two exercises I saw in an article or blog post or YouTube video that look interesting. And if I get to the end of the workout and feel like I've done all I can that day, I'll pack my gym bag and go home.

## MASTER THE HAPPY ENDING

A few rules apply to all end-of-workout training:

### Don't make anything worse

Sore elbow? Not the day for biceps curls and triceps extensions. Tender ankle? No running today. Barking shoulder? Forget that chest-and-back superset you read about at bodybuilding.com. It doesn't matter what you planned to do for metabolic training; if the exercises you chose could make an injury worse, come up with something else.

### Avoid repetitive stress

You'd think I'd be more cognizant of this than most, considering my age (old) and injuries (many). But every now and then I get to the end and realize I have to change things up. For example, on a day you do deadlifts and chin-ups, your forearm muscles could be trashed. That rules out a finisher that depends on grip strength, like heavy carries. If you've done a couple of exercises that exhaust your lower-back muscles—Romanian deadlifts and bent-over rows, say—you might want to avoid any finisher that depends too much on lower-back stability. Or maybe your complex includes an exercise you've just done to exhaustion, like push-ups or shoulder presses. That leads to the final tip.

### Always have a backup plan

One of the big goals of *Supercharged* is to put you in charge, to be your own trainer. It starts with selecting the best exercises to execute Alwyn's plan. But it doesn't stop there. A good trainer knows when to veer off from whatever she planned to do with her client that day. This is especially important if you work out in a commercial gym. Some days it's hard enough to do standard routines with standard equipment. It's doubly, triply, or maybe even quadrupally difficult to do complexes with equipment you can't share for the next 5 to 10 minutes, or to do loaded carries when there's no space to walk in a straight line, with or without a load to carry.

The other type of backup plan is the one I mentioned a couple of times earlier. If you get into your intervals or complexes or Free Zone and realize you have nothing left in the tank, your trainer is obligated to tell you to call it a day. Don't be the kind of trainer who gives the profession a bad name.

## LOADED CARRIES

**BEST FOR:** Basic Training intervals. The key to loaded conditioning is to push yourself to fatigue within the time Alwyn specifies. You can do this by going fast with a light load, or slow with a heavy load.

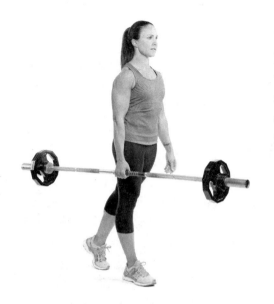

## ✳ Farmer's walk

In Strongman competition, you carry two impossibly heavy things of equally impossible size, one in each hand, at arm's length. But for our purposes, a farmer's walk can be anything you want:

- Two barbells, dumbbells, sandbags, or kettlebells of equal size, one in each hand
- Two unequal weights, alternating sides on each set, or even in the middle of a longer set
- One weight, carried on one side (technically a suitcase walk), alternating as just described

## ✳ Waiter's walk

Same idea, only with one or two weights, of equal or different sizes, carried overhead. One that's particularly challenging: a bottoms-up kettlebell carry.

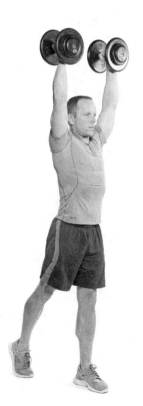
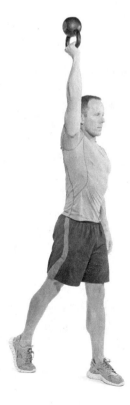

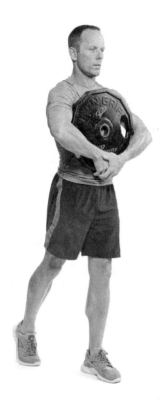

## ✳ Bear-hug walk

Hold a weight plate, sandbag, or non-hyperactive child against your chest. A challenging variation is to hold one or two kettlebells in the rack position, or one or two dumbbells at shoulder height.

## ✳ Pushes or drags

Same concept as the loaded walks: You're pushing or dragging something heavy to build endurance, to push your anaerobic energy systems to their limit, and perhaps to test your fortitude. For between $100 and $200 at elitefts.com or performbetter.com, you can buy a heavy-duty sled that you can load up with weights and push across just about any solid surface. For another $90, you can add a harness that allows you to pull the sled over those same surfaces. Starting around $300, you can get a Prowler, a sled that allows you to push from a more upright position, which will be easier on the back for most of us.

Or you can rig something up at home for yourself, using a wheelbarrow or an actual sled. (You'll want to get your kids' permission before you turn their favorite winter toy into a workout tool.) Or you can push a car up and down your street, if you have an accomplice who'll steer, and who understands what will happen to your face if he hits the brakes without warning.

## LOCOMOTION

**BEST FOR:** the locomotion exercise in Basic Training IV, or intervals in Basic Training I, II, or III. We'll show you two that are kind of fun (if you consider a serious core challenge "fun"). But really, this category can include just about anything that involves forward, backward, sideways, or circular movement. Options include:

- any of the carries, pushes, or drags just described
- the walking lunge, or any traveling variation you can come up with (to the side, in a big circle . . .)
- any of the RAMP exercises in which you move, like carioca or high knees

## ✳ Alligator drag

Get into push-up position with your toes on a pair of sliding discs. Walk forward with your hands, dragging your feet behind you. It's one of the strangest-looking exercises you'll ever do, but a real workout for your core. For $60 you can get a Power Wheel at lifelineusa.com, which is a big wheel with feet straps designed specifically for this type of exercise.

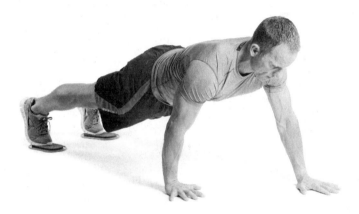

## ✳ Bear crawl

Get down on the floor, your weight on your hands and your toes, torso parallel to the floor, knees bent, back flat. Step forward with your right hand and left leg, without raising your torso any higher. Take the next step with your opposite-side arm and leg. Continue for the designated time.

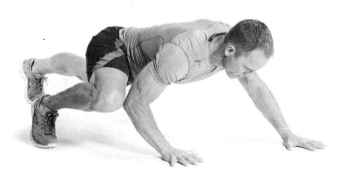

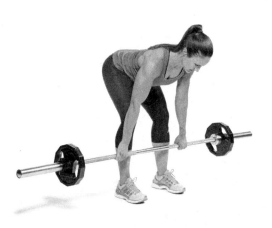

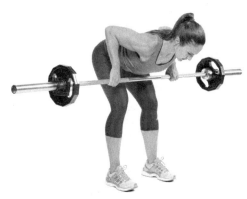

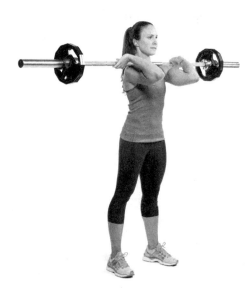

### SUPERCHARGE IT?

The standard bear crawl may be fun for kids, but it's an advanced exercise for adults. You can make it even harder with a twist I read about at wildmantraining.com: Set a ball of some sort on the floor. Get into the bear-crawl position. Bat it forward with one hand, scramble after it, then bat it again with the other hand—all without raising your torso or straightening your legs. You probably want to use a ball that won't roll too far on each smack. Raising one hand off the floor to hit the ball offers a surprising core challenge to an exercise that already has plenty.

## COMPLEXES

**BEST FOR:** Hypertrophy I, II, and III, although you can also use them in the Free Zone in Strength & Power if you like them and want to improve your performance. Some examples:

### ✶ Barbell complexes

Choose a weight that allows you to do all the reps of all three exercises, which means choosing a weight that's appropriate for your weakest lift in the complex, even if it's less challenging for the other lifts. Once you pick up the weight, you'll do all the reps of each exercise, in order, before you set it down.

If you're new to this type of training, try this complex, shown on these pages:

- Bent-over row
- Front squat
- Shoulder press

If you're somewhat more advanced, try this, which includes some exercises we haven't shown yet:

- Romanian deadlift
- High pull
- Clean

Or this:

- Clean
- Front squat
- Push press

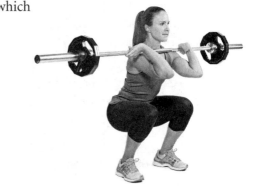

The high pull, clean, and push press are derived from the Olympic clean and jerk. The high pull is a continuation of the jump shrug shown on pages 220–221. The clean is the next step beyond the high pull. The push press uses your lower body to generate momentum to get the bar overhead.

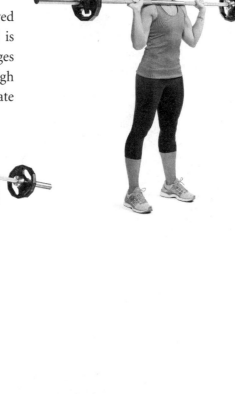

**HIGH PULL**

- Start with the bar at arm's length in front of your thighs.
- Push your hips back slightly and dip your knees, lowering the bar a few inches.
- Execute triple extension: Thrust your hips forward, straighten your knees, and rise up on your toes.
- With the bar moving upward and your arms straight, shrug your shoulders as powerfully as you can, bending your elbows to allow the bar to come up toward your chin. (Word to the wise: Lean your head back at the end. The intersection of bar and chin never ends well for the chin.)

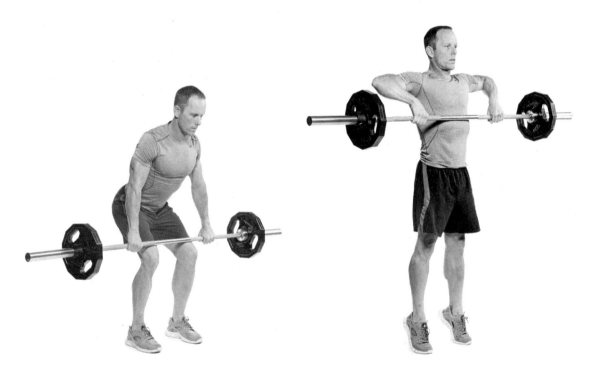

**CLEAN**

- The execution is the same as the high pull, until the bar reaches your upper chest.
- At that point, dip down with your hips and knees.
- At the same time, thrust your elbows forward, taking them below and around the bar. Your goal is to get your upper arms parallel to the floor, with the bar rolled down to your fingertips.
- "Catch" the bar on your shoulders while your hips and knees are bent. With prac-

tice, you'll be able to coordinate it so the bar lands on your shoulders at the bottom of your descent.

- Stand with the weight. You're now in the starting position for the front squat.

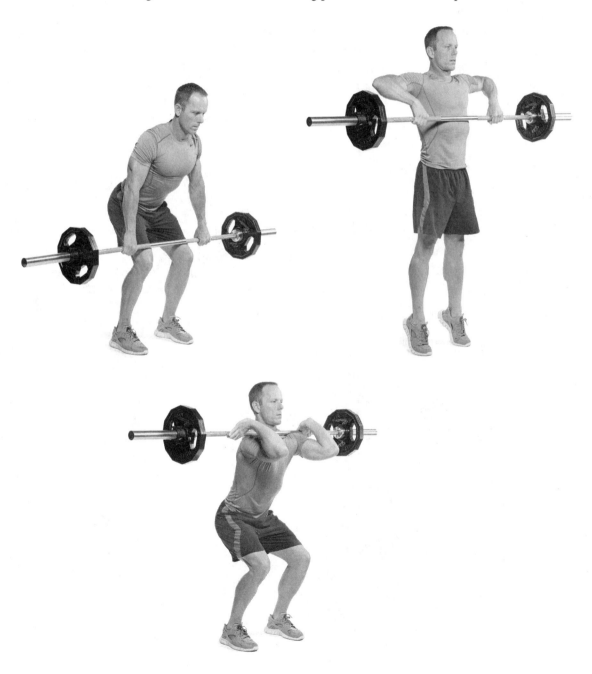

**PUSH PRESS**

- With the bar on your shoulders following your front squats, lower your elbows and roll the bar down to your palms, gripping it with your thumbs under and fingers over the bar.
- Dip your hips and knees, and press the bar overhead as you straighten them. (Again, remember to get your chin out of the way.)
- You want your momentum to get the bar about a third of the way up, and then use your shoulders and arms to press it the rest of the way.

## ✳ Dumbbell complexes

With two dumbbells, try this:

- Two-point row (aka bent-over row)
- High pull (like the barbell version described earlier, although it'll look more like an upright row; stop when the weights reach your lower chest)
- Shoulder press (or, if you're feeling adventurous, a squat and press)

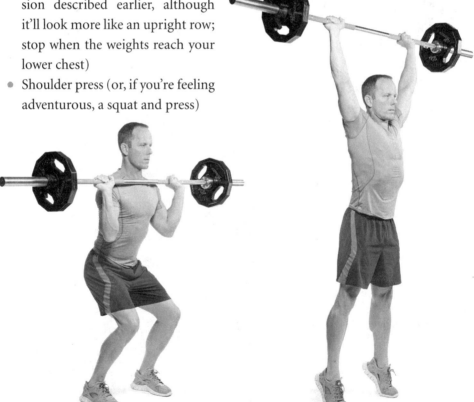

## Clean Power Generation

Lifters with experience using the clean, high pull, and push press may wonder why we have these exercises here, at the end of workouts in Hypertrophy, rather than in the power category at the beginning of workouts in Basic Training. I asked Alwyn the same question.

First off, he thinks the power clean is among the best power exercises you can do. It's a more advanced version of the exercise shown here, with the weight starting on the floor, like a deadlift. But the benefits only accrue with a combination of perfect technique and high intensity. Perfect technique takes a long time to learn (I'm still working on mine), and you don't want to try heavy loads until you've achieved it. Alwyn wants readers to push themselves on the power exercises in Basic Training. You won't lose any benefits by using simpler exercises.

In the context of metabolic training, however, technique is less crucial. You aren't going to hurt yourself if you mistime your catch and the bar hits the top of your chest instead of sticking a perfect landing on your front deltoids.

All that said, if you're confident in your technique, you can use the clean, high pull, or push press (or any other Olympic variation you've mastered) in Basic Training. But if all you know about them is what you just learned in this chapter, please stick with the power exercises in Chapter 15.

Or this:

- Romanian deadlift
- Clean (pull the weights up explosively and catch them so the ends of the dumbbells rest on top of your shoulders)
- Front squat (starting from the catch position of the dumbbell clean)

## ✴ Mixed complex

- Body-weight squat
- Standing row with one or two bands
- Push-up

## FREE ZONE

**BEST FOR:** finishing up Strength I, II, and III. Alwyn's rules, as described, are simple enough:

- Pick two exercises.
- Do 8 to 10 reps of each without rest in between.
- Do as many sets as you can in 5 minutes.

But let me throw in some caveats, wrinkles, and exceptions, based on how I ended up using these exercises in my own workouts:

- For a bigger metabolic boost, choose two unilateral exercises. So, for example, you could do a one-arm cable row and a one-arm cable chest press, as shown in chapters 10 and 11. If you do 8 reps of each exercise with each arm, that's 32 reps per set. You're also bracing your core the whole time, adding an extra 5 minutes of core training to your program.
- Another way to use the same concept: kneeling or half-kneeling single-arm biceps curls and triceps extensions. Kneel on a padded surface (if you use a thick Airex

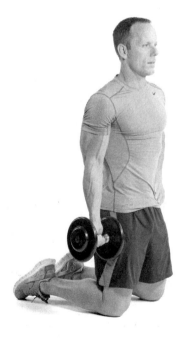
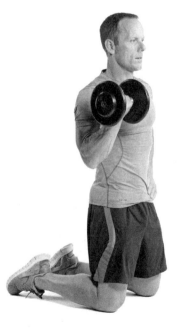

pad, you add an instability challenge for your core) holding the weight in your right hand. Do 8 to 10 curls, switch arms, and repeat. Then do the same with overhead triceps extensions. Keep your torso upright and shoulders and hips square.

- Another option is to do a single combination exercise (like a squat and press). Doing as many sets as possible in 5 minutes is one hell of a metabolic and muscular challenge.
- You can make up your own combination exercise. One I learned at the 2012 Fitness Summit in Kansas City:
  ○ Clean the weight to your shoulders.
  ○ Do a reverse lunge (shown on page 149) with each leg.
  ○ That's one rep. Only 7 to 9 more to finish the set!
- You can do a single locomotion exercise (carries, bear crawls, sled pushes or drags . . .) for a defined distance that takes 15 to 20 seconds. Travel that distance as many times as you can in 5 minutes.
- Complexes are also allowed. Again, do as many as you can in 5 minutes (choosing your own rep range for each exercise), rather than resting a specified amount of time in between.

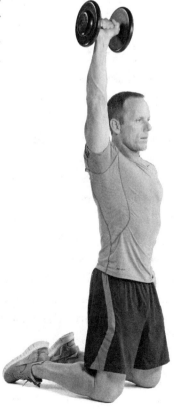
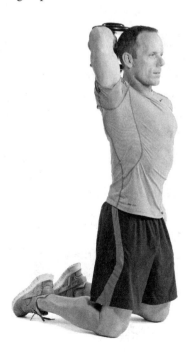

# 17

# RAMP It Up, Tone It Down

I CAN'T PROMISE THAT A WORKOUT you begin well will also end well. All I know from my own experience is that the better the warm-up, the better you'll do in the middle, the part that matters most. You'll lift more, and lift better, when your muscles and joints are warm, when their movement is smooth and unobstructed, and when your body supplies you with a biologically active dose of adrenaline, the secret sauce that quickens your heart rate, widens your blood vessels, shovels fuel into your muscles, speeds up your muscles' contraction rate, and does what you expect any good stimulant to do. That is, it stimulates you to do more than you would attempt if you weren't amped up.

That's what a good warm-up accomplishes, and Alwyn's RAMP protocol is a very good warm-up. As you may remember, the acronym stands for *Range of motion, Activation,* and *Movement Preparation.*

*Range of motion* refers specifically to joint mobility. I like to think of these exercises as kind of a pre-workout checkup. If something is tighter than it should be, you'll discover it here. This is one part of the program when it's perfectly fine to invest more time and attention on a problem area.

*Activation* is a different but synergistic idea. You're waking up your muscles, getting them ready not just for the specific movement patterns—the squats, deadlifts, pushes, pulls, and lunges—but for lifting in general. It's like your muscles are getting their buzz on.

*Movement prep* gets your body ready to act and react in a coordinated, athletic way, with all limbs in all directions.

Ten minutes of RAMP will raise your core temperature—the most literal aspect of warming up—and increase blood flow into the specific muscles you're about to use. The faster exercises at the end will ensure a dose of adrenaline by the time you're ready to lift.

The exercises are presented in a prescriptive way, with reps or duration. But this part of the system is also flexible. If you have rehab exercises you need to perform, or corrective drills you like to do before lifting, you can add them to RAMP. Personally, I like to start my workout with the recovery exercises in the second half of this chapter. And sometimes, when I'm feeling especially middle-aged, I'll throw in some basic, old-fashioned stretches for problem areas. The whole routine might take me 20 minutes instead of the standard 10. But when the alternative is a compromised workout with higher injury risk, I'd rather invest the time up front than pay for poor results later.

## RAMP

| RAMP • Use at the start of each A and B workout | |
|---|---|
| **Exercise** | **Reps/distance** |
| Half-kneeling hip-flexor stretch | 30 seconds each side |
| Half-kneeling thoracic rotation | 10 each side |
| Hip raise (or) Single-leg hip raise | 10 8 each side |
| Spiderman climb | 5 each side |
| Spiderman climb with reach | 5 each side |
| Squat to stand | 10 |
| Reverse lunge with reach and twist | 5 each side |
| Side lunge with touch | 5 each side |
| Cossack lunge | 5 each side |
| Jog | 2 runs of 10–20 yards, or 20–40 steps in place |
| Side shuffle | 2 runs of 10–20 yards |
| High-knee run | 1 run of 10–20 yards, or 10–20 high-knee steps in place |
| Carioca | 2 runs of 10–20 yards, or 20 crossover jumping jacks |

## ✳ Half-kneeling hip-flexor stretch

- Kneel on a pad on your right knee, with your left foot flat on the floor in front of you and your knee bent.
- Straighten your torso, and put your hands either on your hips or behind your head.
- Shift your weight forward, keeping your torso upright, until you feel a stretch on the right side of your pelvis.
- Hold for 30 seconds.
- Switch sides and repeat.
- Go for a gentle stretch here; you can get more aggressive in subsequent exercises.

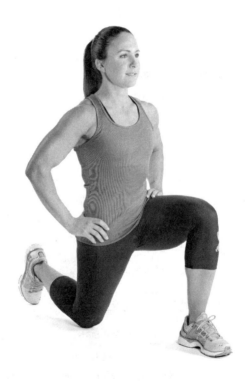

# ✳ Half-kneeling thoracic rotation

- Kneel on a pad on your right knee, with your left foot flat on the floor in front of you and your knee bent.
- Bend forward at the hips and set your right hand on the floor directly beneath your shoulder (about 15 inches from your left foot).
- Reach up and back with your left arm, following it with your eyes, until both arms are perpendicular to the floor.
- Sweep your left arm down and past your left leg, reaching under your right arm. That's one rep.
- Do all your reps, switch sides, and repeat.
- You aren't looking for a big upper-torso stretch here. You'll have several chances to extend your range of motion.

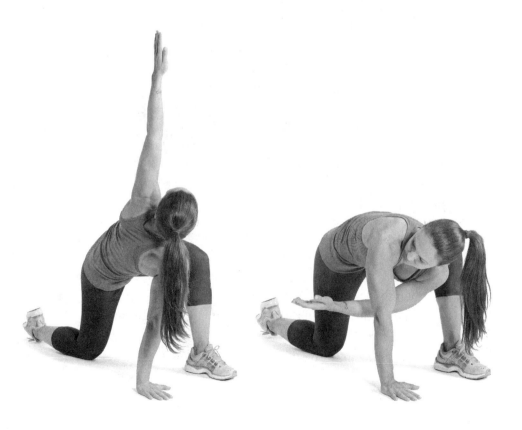

## ✳ Hip raise

- Lie on your back on the floor, with your knees bent, heels on the floor, and arms out to your sides.
- Push down through your heels and lift your hips off the floor as high as you can, feeling the contraction in your glutes and hamstrings (but not in your lower back).
- Lower your hips close to the floor, and repeat.
- You can also do this with one leg at a time, as shown. Lift the foot of the nonworking leg off the floor.

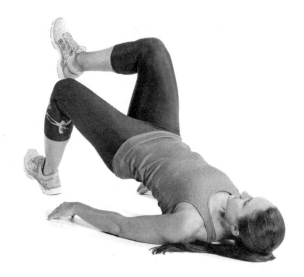

## ✳ Spiderman climb

- Set up in push-up position.
- Lift your right foot up next to your right hand.
- As you set your foot down, drop your hips *slightly* to feel the stretch in your lower abdomen and hip flexors.
- Move your right foot back to the starting position, then lift your left foot up next to your left hand.
- Continue alternating until you finish the set.

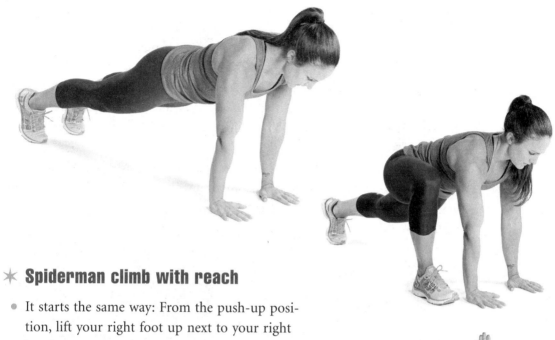

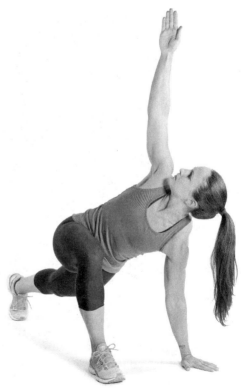

## ✳ **Spiderman climb with reach**

- It starts the same way: From the push-up position, lift your right foot up next to your right hand.
- Reach up and back with your right hand, following your hand with your eyes, until your arms are perpendicular to the floor.
- Lower your hand, move your foot back to the starting position, and repeat on the other side.
- Alternate until you finish the set.
- Yes, it's like the half-kneeling thoracic rotation, only now your lower back and pelvis turn as a unit with your shoulders, adding a mild stabilization and coordination challenge to the movement. You should feel the stretch all the way down the arm that's overhead, starting with the biceps and going through your chest, abdomen, and the inner thigh of the opposite-side leg.

## ✳ Squat to stand

- Stand with your hands at your sides and your feet shoulder-width apart.
- Bend at the hips, keeping your legs straight, and reach toward your toes.
- Push your hips back, bend your knees, and descend into a squat, grabbing your toes whenever you can and pulling yourself down into the deepest squat you can manage. Keep your arms straight and just inside your knees, with your feet flat on the floor.
- Pull your shoulders and head back as you tighten your entire upper body.
- Hold on to your toes as you bend forward again, lifting your hips and straightening your legs. You should feel a deep stretch in your hamstrings.
- Return to the starting position and repeat.

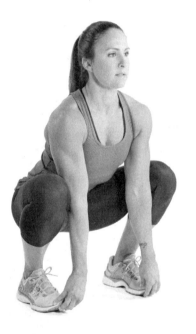 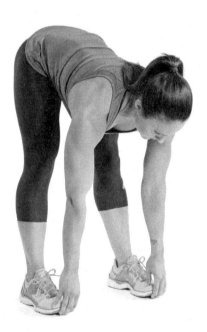

## ✳ Reverse lunge with reach

- Stand with your feet hip-width apart.
- Take a long step back into a reverse lunge with your left leg.
- Bend to the left while reaching overhead with your right hand.
- At the same time, turn your shoulders to the right and reach toward your left foot with your right hand.

- You should feel a nice stretch all the way down your left side: triceps, lats, obliques, hip flexors.
- Return to the starting position, and repeat with your left leg stepping back, leaning and turning to your left.
- Alternate until you finish the set.
- Women: Feel free to look lovely and graceful while doing this one. Men: Remember that everyone in the gym is looking at either themselves or the lovely and graceful women. No one's looking at you.

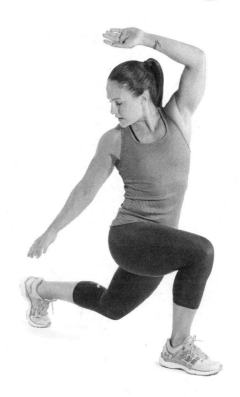

## ✴ Side lunge with touch

- Stand with your feet hip-width apart.
- Take a long step to your left and descend into a side lunge.
- Touch the floor with both hands, one on either side of your left foot.
- Return to the starting position and repeat to your right.
- Alternate until you finish the set.
- You're looking for a fairly deep stretch along the insides of the extended leg, through your pelvic floor.

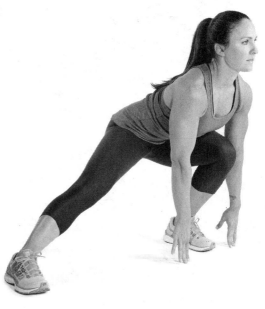

## ✳ Cossack lunge

- Stand with legs akimbo (a phrase I've waited most of my career to type). That is, stand with your legs wide apart, knees bent, toes turned out—like the horse stance in karate, only not quite that low or threatening.
- Keeping your torso upright, lean to your left, raising the toes of your right foot.
- Shift to the right, raising the toes of your left foot.
- Alternate sides, going a little deeper each time. It's okay to do extra reps if it takes more than 5 to achieve your full range of motion.
- You should feel the stretch all the way up your extended leg, from the calf through the hamstrings, up to your lower abdomen, and over to the inner-thigh muscles of the leg that's bent.

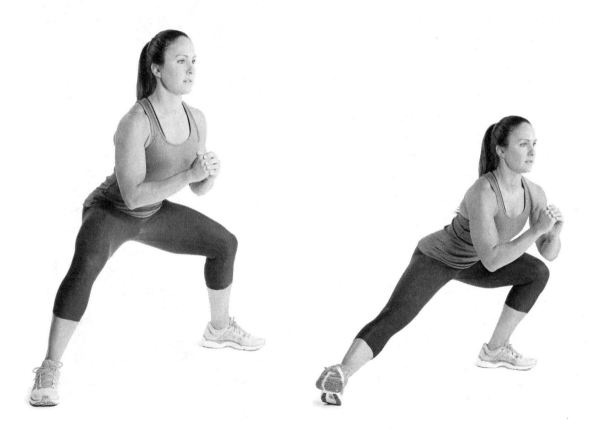

## ✳ Jog

This is just like it sounds: If you can't jog 10 to 20 yards and back, jog in place for 20 to 40 steps.

## ✳ Side shuffle

- Stand sideways to an open stretch of floor, with your left side toward your direction of travel.
- Get into an athletic position with your feet wider than your shoulders, knees bent slightly, torso leaning forward, arms out to your sides. It should look like you're guarding someone in basketball.
- Slide your right foot until it touches your left.
- Immediately step to the left with your left foot, and slide your right foot to meet it.
- Continue for 10 to 20 yards, stop, catch your breath, and repeat by sliding to your right.

No open space? Try this alternative:

- Shuffle twice to your left, then reach and touch the floor outside your left foot with your right hand.
- Shuffle twice to your right, reaching and touching the floor outside your right foot with your left hand.
- Do 10 to each side.

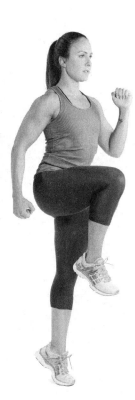

## ✳ High-knee run

- Stand facing the open space, with your feet hip-width apart, arms at your sides, and elbows bent.
- Run forward, lifting your knee as high as possible on each step while swinging the opposite-side arm forward and the same-side arm backward.
- Take very short steps, landing on the balls of your feet each time and pushing off immediately.

No space? This one's easy to do in place, since even with a track you're hardly moving forward on each step.

## ✳ Carioca

This is a lateral-movement drill in which your trailing leg alternately crosses behind and in front of your leading leg. Those of us who learned it while playing sports are at a slight advantage, in that our bodies kinda-sorta remember how to do it. Others will have to practice it a few times before it feels natural.

- As with the side shuffle, stand with your left side toward open space, your feet shoulder-width apart and arms relaxed.
- Swing your right foot behind and past your left foot.
- Take a long step to the left with your left foot.
- Swing your right foot in front of and past your left foot.
- Take a long step to the left with your left foot.
- Repeat until you've gone 10 to 20 yards, stop, catch your breath, and repeat, this time moving to your right.

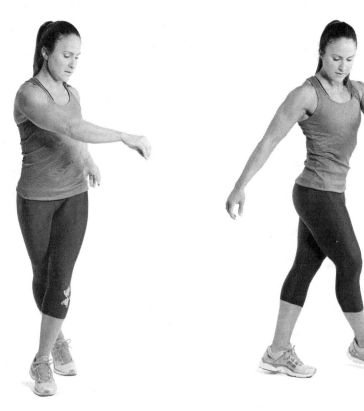

- Speed it up as soon as you get the hang of it. When you go fast, your hips rotate rapidly, and your shoulders turn with your hips.

No space? This one is even harder to replicate than the side shuffle. The closest we can come is the crossover jumping jack:

- Stand with your feet together, arms at your sides.
- Jump out to the sides with both feet as your arms come together above your head.
- Instead of bringing your feet together as your arms come down, cross them in front of and behind each other, alternating on each rep.
- You can also cross your arms in front instead of lifting them overhead, although I think I speak for lots of us when I say that may be one coordination challenge too many.

## RECOVERY

If we think about recovery at all, most of us assume it happens outside the gym, in the days between workouts. And that's a perfectly legitimate way to look at recovery in general. We know our muscles synthesize protein at an accelerated rate for 24 to 48 hours post-workout. We know our connective tissues need more time than muscles to repair themselves, since they have a smaller blood supply and thus fewer nutrients flowing in and out. Even our nervous system needs downtime after ramping up for a productive training session.

But the smart play is to begin preparing for your next workout before you leave the weight room, with stretches and the foam-rolling exercises shown on these pages. Stretches take advantage of your body's elevated temperature, allowing you to restore their length and reduce some of the tension induced by your workout. Foam rolling works out the kinks, breaking up the small knots and adhesions that accumulate when you lift aggressively.

You can pick up a 6-inch-thick foam roller at a sporting-goods store or online at performbetter.com, as I mentioned in Chapter 7. How you use it is really up to you. You can try the exercises here, in this sequence, for starters, and then add or subtract to suit your own body.

I highly recommend spending more time on problem areas. Every surface you roll over will feel like a problem area at first, but after a few sessions you'll get a feel for which muscles need more work. Look for tender or more sensitive spots, and roll over them a few more times than you do tissue that feels normal.

Alwyn's basic guidelines for tissue recovery and maintenance:

- Spend about 10 to 20 seconds on muscles that don't have any obvious problems.
- When you stretch, hold each one about 30 seconds. Again, you're encouraged to take more time with muscles that are shorter or tighter on one side than the other.
- Several of the RAMP exercises, especially the lunges and reaches, make perfectly fine stretches. Just hold the final position instead of moving into and out of it.
- Roll or stretch muscles from top to bottom or bottom to top, along the same direction as the muscle bellies. If a muscle goes north and south, don't try to work it east to west.
- You can stretch or foam roll just about any time you want: before or after workouts, on days in between, even multiple times a day if you think you need it. Just be smart about it. Don't stretch first thing in the morning, when your spinal discs have more fluid and are more vulnerable to rupture. Don't do an aggressive stretch after an extended period at your desk or on the road.
- Pay attention to your feet and calves. A few minutes of rolling a tennis ball around the soles of your feet will tend to improve your overall lower-body range of motion. It's something you can do while sitting at your desk or talking on the phone. Same with stretching out your calves. Point your toes as far as you can, then pull your toes up toward your shins.
- While you're sitting at your desk, remember to get up and move around a few times an hour. Sitting distorts posture and cuts off circulation.

## RECOVERY EXERCISES

### ✴ Glute roll

- The fibers of the gluteus maximus run east and west, perpendicular to those of your hamstrings and quadriceps. That's why you want to position the roller as shown, so you can roll sideways, rather than back and forth.
- Sit on the roll with one cheek, with your targeted leg crossed over your nonworking leg, and roll from left to right and right to left.

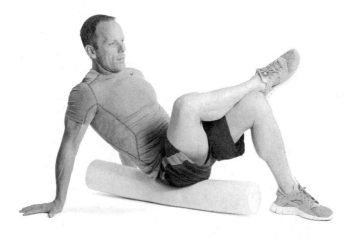

## ✳ Calf roll

- Set the roll under one calf, and cross the ankle of your nonworking leg over that shin to increase pressure.
- Lift your hips up, supporting your weight on your hands, and pull and push your calf muscles over the roll from ankle to knee.
- Switch legs and repeat.

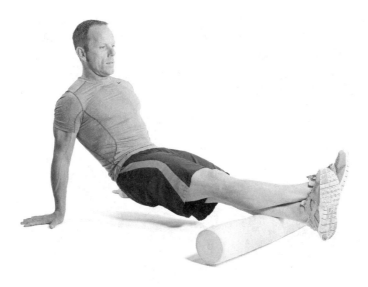

## ✳ Ham roll

- Same technique as the calf roll, rolling one leg at a time, from the bottom of your knee to the gluteal crease.
- Some prefer to roll both legs at the same time.

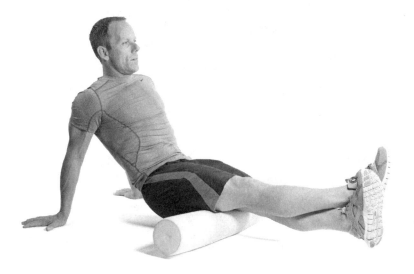

## ✳ Quad roll

- Lie facedown, with your front thigh on the roll and your weight distributed between your forearms and the nonworking leg, which rests on the floor.
- Pull yourself over the roll, hitting everything from the top of your knee to your groin.

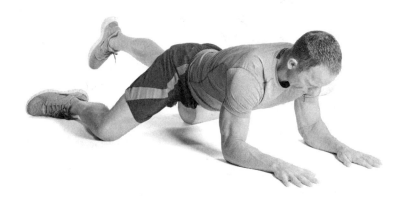

## ✳ IT-band roll

- Lie on your side, with the outside of your thigh on the roll and your weight on one hand.
- Pull and push yourself over the roll from your hip to the top of your knee.
- To take some pressure off, you can place the foot of your non-rolling leg on the floor.

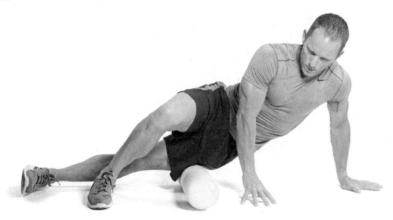

## ✳ Adductor roll

- Lie facedown, with your inner thigh over the roller. The roller itself will be at an odd angle that takes some adjustment to get right. It's basically perpendicular to your working leg, and at about a 45-degree angle to your torso.
- The nonworking leg is flat on the floor. Your weight is supported on it and your forearms.
- Roll from the inside top of your knee as high as you dare.

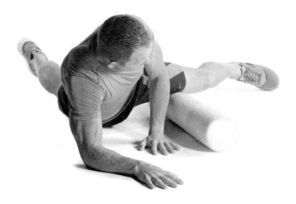

# PART 4

# THE PROGRAMS

# 18

# How to Train

Two TYPES OF READERS WILL BE utterly confused when they read this introduction to the programs. One type will start here, skipping all the chapters that explain how Alwyn's template system works, and how to choose exercises that are appropriate for you. They'll be utterly confused by the blank spaces on the template where they were expecting to see exercises. Another type will read everything *but* this chapter, and only come back to read it when they get to the gym and realize their workouts don't work.

So, with apologies to the readers who started at the beginning and who understand exactly how we got here (and are understandably impatient to get started), here's what you need to know:

1. Alwyn's system includes ten programs: Basic Training I–IV, Hypertrophy I–III, and Strength & Power I–III.
2. You must choose a starting program. I hope most of you will begin with Basic Training I, but some should start elsewhere, as I explain in Chapter 7. And I know some of you will roll the dice and start with whichever program looks most in-

teresting to you. Frankly, if I hadn't written the book, I might do the same thing. But since I did write it, I hope you'll follow the Chapter 7 advice.

3. Each program in Basic Training and Hypertrophy includes two workouts: A and B. Same with Strength & Power I. Strength & Power II and III have A, B, C, and D workouts.

4. Each workout in every program begins with RAMP, Alwyn's warm-up protocol. Please do the exercises as shown and described in Chapter 17 when you're starting out, although it's perfectly fine to add or substitute exercises if you know what you're doing and have good reason to personalize your routine.

5. You need to choose your own exercises for the next four parts of each workout: core (Chapter 14), power and/or combination (Chapter 15), strength (Chapters 8 through 13, one for each of the six movement patterns), and metabolic training (Chapter 16).

6. Each of those chapters offers advice on where to begin with each movement pattern or type of training. You don't have to reread each chapter in its entirety; just look for the starting point that makes the most sense for you; for many readers it will be the very first exercise. Fill that exercise in on the template, and move on to the next.

7. Our goal in *Supercharged* is for each reader to create a customized workout system to fit your abilities and ambitions. Chapter 22 shows a sample of how one person (me) might choose exercises for each workout in each program. If you're okay with my choices, you can simply photocopy those, or copy them onto the workout logs you download from werkit.com.

What follows is divided into three parts:

- A look at a sample template (from Basic Training I)
- A quick explanation of how the workouts work
- Lists of the exercises in each category

Those of you who're familiar with Alwyn's NROL programs (especially those who read *NROL for Life*) can skim over this.

## BASIC TRAINING I

| Workout A | | | | | |
| --- | --- | --- | --- | --- | --- |
| Category/exercise | Sets/reps | Workout 1 | Workout 2 | Workout 3 | Workout 4 |
| *Core* | | | | | |
| Stability | 1–2 x 30 seconds | | | | |
| Dynamic Stability | 1–2 x 10 | | | | |
| *Power* | | | | | |
| | 2 x 5 | | | | |
| *Strength* | | | | | |
| 1a: Squat | 1–2 x 15 | | | | |
| 1b: Pull | 1–2 x 15 | | | | |
| 2a: Single-leg stance | 1–2 x 15 | | | | |
| 2b: Push | 1–2 x 15 | | | | |
| *Metabolic* | | | | | |
| | 2–4 x 1 minute work/ 2 minutes recovery | | | | |

For those new to NROL-style training, here's a quick primer:

## CATEGORY/EXERCISE

This is where you fill in an exercise from the specified category. So for "stability," you select an exercise shown in that section in Chapter 14.

## SETS/REPS

*Rep* is short for *repetition*, a single execution of an exercise. One push-up is one repetition. A *set* is the number of consecutive repetitions of that exercise Alwyn wants you to do in this workout. If the template shows "1–2 x 15," that means 1 or 2 sets of 15 reps. Remember, 15 reps is a goal. You may not reach it every time. Whether you do or don't, *it shouldn't be easy to hit the target.* If it is, you need to increase the weight or difficulty for the next set (if you're doing multiple sets) or the next workout (if you're only doing one set).

## WORKOUT 1, WORKOUT 2 . . .

These are the columns you use to fill in the weight you use and the number of repetitions you complete (or the time you hold a core-stability exercise). The first time you do each workout, you'll fill in the column for Workout 1. The second time you'll use the column for Workout 2. Here's how you might fill it in:

| Category/exercise | Sets/reps | Workout 1 | Workout 2 | Workout 3 | Workout 4 |
|---|---|---|---|---|---|
| 1a: Goblet squat | 1–2 x 15 | 25/15<br>25/13 | 25/15<br>30/12 | | |

In this example, you select the goblet squat (the Level 2 exercise for that movement pattern). In Workout 1, you get 15 reps with 25 pounds on the first set, and 13 on the second. Because you didn't get 15 on both, you decide to use the same weight for Workout 2. This time you feel stronger on the first set, and it's slightly easier to get all 15 reps. So you use 30 pounds on the second set. Since you only get 12 reps, that's your weight for Workout 3, when you'll try to get 15 for at least one set, if not both.

Keep in mind that you're doing another workout—Workout B—in between. So if you do Workout A for the first time on Monday, you'd do Workout B on Wednesday. Then you'd repeat Workout A on Friday. The next week it would be the opposite: B on Monday, A on Wednesday, and B again on Friday.

## 1a, 1b, 2a, 2b

These designations in front of the strength exercises indicate *alternating sets.* You do the 1a exercise, rest long enough to catch your breath, do 1b, rest, and repeat until you've completed all your sets of both exercises. Then you move on to 2a and 2b. (Sometimes there's also a "c" exercise, but it doesn't change the system. Do a set of 1a, rest, 1b, rest, 1c, rest, and then repeat until you finish all your sets.)

## "Wait, *How* Long Do I Rest?"

In the first three NROL books Alwyn specified rest periods between sets, usually 30, 60, or 90 seconds. In *Life* we made a more general suggestion: Rest just long enough to catch your breath and recover your strength. But some readers told me, via the NROL forums at jpfitness.com, that they prefer specifics.

So here they are:

### Core Training

If you're doing two core exercises in a workout, try not to rest in between. Do the first one, then do the second as soon as you can (some require a bit of setup). If you do a second set of each exercise, rest about 45 seconds before you begin those sets. When the workout calls for multiple sets of one core exercise, rest about 45 seconds between sets.

### Power and Combination Exercises

Rest 60 seconds between sets, or longer if you need it. You don't want to do either type of exercise in a state of incomplete recovery. Put another way, you don't want fatigue to diminish your performance, and thus compromise your results.

### Strength Exercises

The general guidelines:

- For high-rep sets (12 or more per set), 30 seconds is usually enough. The exception is when you're doing single-limb exercises. Fifteen lunges with each leg should require more than 30 seconds to recover.
- For medium-rep sets (8 to 10), 60 seconds works most of the time.
- For low-rep sets (4 to 6), Alwyn typically suggests 90 seconds. But if you don't need 90 seconds, don't feel obligated to take it. You'll know you didn't take enough time if your performance on your next set is substantially worse.

All this said, I hope you'll use your own judgment as you get comfortable with the system. If it feels like too much time between sets, you can work a little faster. If it feels like too little, you can slow it down. Just avoid these two extremes:

*You never rest between sets, and your workout turns into a glorified Pump & Tone class.*

This is anaerobic training. It only works if you use your anaerobic energy systems. You should need some recovery between sets. If you don't, you aren't working hard enough to get the results you want. You want your muscles to reach a state of fatigue by the end of almost every set in this program. That doesn't mean *extreme* fatigue, the kind you get when you force your muscles to complete 2 or 3 more reps after it's clear they've reached the point of momentary exhaustion. But almost every set should at least be difficult enough to force you to stop and catch your breath.

*You screw around too long between sets, and rarely work up a sweat.*

You want to be strong for each set. Otherwise, you won't be able to impose enough mechanical tension or produce enough muscle damage to get stronger and develop new muscle tissue (or at least improve the quality of what you have now). That's crucial to your success. But Alwyn's workouts are also designed to produce metabolic stress. That comes from accumulated fatigue.

# THE EXERCISES

## Core: stabilization

| Level | Exercise | Goal |
|---|---|---|
| Level 1 | Plank | AE |
| | Side plank | ALF |
| | Cable tall kneeling static hold | AR |
| Level 2 | Plank with reduced base of support | AE |
| | Side plank with reduced base of support | ALF |
| | Cable half-kneeling static hold | AR |
| Level 3 | Feet-elevated plank | AE |
| | Feet-elevated side plank | ALF |
| Level 4 | Feet-elevated push-up hold with reduced base of support | AE |
| | Feet-elevated side plank with reduced base of support | ALF |
| Level 5 | Feet-elevated plank with unstable point of contact | AE |
| | Swiss-ball side plank | ALF |

## Core: dynamic stabilization

| Level | Exercise | Goal |
|---|---|---|
| Level 1 | Plank and pulldown | AE |
|  | Side plank and row | ALF |
| Level 2 | Push-away | AE |
|  | Mountain climber | HF |
| Level 3 | Swiss-ball rollout | AE |
|  | Cable tall kneeling chop | AR |
|  | Swiss-ball mountain climber | HF |
| Level 4 | Suspended fallout | AE |
|  | Cable half-kneeling chop | AR |
|  | Swiss-ball jackknife | HF |
| Level 5 | Suspended jackknife and push-up | HF |
|  | Cable chop and reverse lunge | AR |
|  | Turkish get-up | ALF |
| Level 5 progression | Cable horizontal chop |  |

AE: anti-extension
ALF: anti-lateral flexion
AR: anti-rotation
HF: hip flexion

## Combination

| Level | Exercise | Notes |
|---|---|---|
| Level 1 | Reverse lunge and shoulder press |  |
| Level 2 | Romanian deadlift and row |  |
| Level 3 | Squat and press |  |
| Level 4 | Push-up and one-arm row |  |
| Level 5 | Offset squat and one-arm shoulder press |  |

## Power

| Level | Exercise | Notes |
|---|---|---|
| Level 1 | Box jump | |
| Level 2 | Jump squat | |
| Level 3, option 1 | Kettlebell swing | Double- or single-arm |
| Level 3, option 2 | Explosive push-up | |
| Level 4 | Jump shrug | |
| Level 5 | Dumbbell single-arm snatch | |

## Squat

| Level | Exercise | Notes |
|---|---|---|
| Level 1 | Body-weight squat | |
| Level 2 | Goblet squat | Use dumbbell, kettlebell, or weight plate |
| Level 2.5 | Kettlebell rack-position squat | |
| Level 3 | Front squat | |
| Level 3.5 | Offset overhead squat | |
| Level 4 | Back squat<br>(or)<br>Hex-bar deadlift | |
| Level 5 | Overhead squat | |

## Hinge

| Level | Exercise | Notes |
|-------|----------|-------|
| Level 1 | Swiss-ball supine hip extension | |
| Level 1.5 | Supine hip extension with leg curl | |
| Level 2 | Romanian deadlift<br>(or)<br>Cable pull-through<br>(or)<br>Kettlebell or dumbbell sumo deadlift | |
| Level 3 | Rack deadlift | |
| Level 4 | Deadlift<br>(or)<br>Sumo deadlift<br>(or)<br>Hex-bar deadlift | |
| Level 5 | Wide-grip deadlift | |

## Push

| Level | Exercise | Direction of push |
|-------|----------|-------------------|
| Modified Level 1 | Push-up with hands elevated | Horizontal |
| Level 1 | Push-up<br>(or)<br>Jackknife push-up | Horizontal<br><br>Vertical |
| Level 2 | Standing single-arm cable chest press | Horizontal |
| Level 2.5 | Push-up with hands suspended | Horizontal |
| Level 3 | T push-up<br>(or)<br>T push-up with weights | Horizontal |
| Level 4 | Dumbbell bench press | Horizontal |
| Level 4.1 | Dumbbell single-arm bench press | Horizontal |
| Level 5 | Dumbbell shoulder press<br>(or)<br>Dumbbell alternating shoulder press | Vertical |
| Level 7.5 | Barbell bench press | Horizontal |

## Pull

| Level | Exercise | Direction of pull |
|---|---|---|
| Level 1 | Standing cable row | Horizontal |
| Level 2 | Kneeling lat pulldown | Vertical |
| Level 3 | Dumbbell two-point row (or) Dumbbell three-point row (or) Dumbbell chest-supported row | Horizontal |
| Level 4 | Inverted row | Horizontal |
| Level 4.5 | Suspended row | Horizontal |
| Level 5 | Chin-up | Vertical |

## Lunge

| Level | Exercise | Notes |
|---|---|---|
| Level 1 | Split squat | |
| Level 2 | Reverse lunge | |
| Level 2.5 | Side lunge | |
| Level 3 | Split squat, rear foot elevated | |
| Level 4 | Forward lunge | |
| Level 5 | Walking lunge | |

## Single-leg stance

| Level | Exercise | Notes |
|---|---|---|
| Level 1 | Step-up | |
| Level 2 | Offset-loaded step-up | |
| Level 2.25 | Crossover step-up | |
| Level 2.75 | Overhead step-up | |
| Level 3 | Single-leg Romanian deadlift | |
| Level 4 | Single-leg squat | |
| Level 5 | Single-leg deadlift | |

# 19

# Basic Training

QUICK REMINDERS:

- Most readers should start the program with Basic Training I. Some, however (particularly those who recently completed the programs in *NROL for Life*), should start with Basic Training IV. See Chapter 7 for details.
- Most readers should do each workout (A and B) in each program (Basic Training I, II, III, and IV) six times before moving on to the next program. More advanced lifters, especially those who've done Alwyn's programs from previous books, should do each workout four times.
- Before you begin, select exercises from the lists on the previous pages.
- Many readers can simply begin Basic Training I with the first exercise in each category (the one labeled Level 1). Those with more experience should start with the first exercise that will challenge them. Alwyn starts you out with sets of 15 repetitions. Even advanced lifters can get great workouts in Basic Training I using some of this book's Level 1 and Level 2 exercises. If nothing else, your body will

appreciate a break from a steady diet of barbell squats, deadlifts, and bench presses.

- When possible, use the same exercises throughout each Basic Training program, and then switch exercises when you begin the next program. The core category is a big exception. As soon as you master a variation, or run out of ways to make it challenging, move up to the next one, following the guidelines in Chapter 14.
- Start each workout with Alwyn's RAMP program, shown in Chapter 17.
- Finish each workout with recovery exercises (also shown in Chapter 17).

## BASIC TRAINING I

| Workout A | | | | | |
|---|---|---|---|---|---|
| Category/exercise | Sets/reps | Workout 1 | Workout 2 | Workout 3 | Workout 4 |
| *Core* | | | | | |
| Stability | 1–2 x 30 seconds | | | | |
| Dynamic Stability | 1–2 x 10 | | | | |
| *Power* | | | | | |
| | 2 x 5 | | | | |
| *Strength* | | | | | |
| 1a: Squat | 1–2 x 15 | | | | |
| 1b: Pull | 1–2 x 15 | | | | |
| 2a: Single-leg stance | 1–2 x 15 | | | | |
| 2b: Push | 1–2 x 15 | | | | |
| *Intervals* | | | | | |
| | 2–4 x 1 minute work/ 2 minutes recovery | | | | |

**Workout B**

| Category/exercise | Sets/reps | Workout 1 | Workout 2 | Workout 3 | Workout 4 |
|---|---|---|---|---|---|
| *Core* | | | | | |
| Stability | 1–2 x 30 seconds | | | | |
| Dynamic stability | 2 x 10 | | | | |
| *Combination* | | | | | |
| | 2 x 5–8 | | | | |
| *Strength* | | | | | |
| 1a: Hinge | 1–2 x 15 | | | | |
| 1b: Push | 1–2 x 15 | | | | |
| 2a: Lunge | 1–2 x 15 | | | | |
| 2b: Pull | 1–2 x 15 | | | | |
| *Intervals* | | | | | |
| | 2–4 x 1 minute work/ 2 minutes recovery | | | | |

# BASIC TRAINING II

**Workout A**

| Category/exercise | Sets/reps | Workout 1 | Workout 2 | Workout 3 | Workout 4 |
|---|---|---|---|---|---|
| *Core* | | | | | |
| Stability | 2 x 30 seconds | | | | |
| *Combination* | | | | | |
| | 2 x 10 | | | | |
| *Strength* | | | | | |
| 1a: Lunge | 2–4 x 10 | | | | |
| 1b: Pull | 2–4 x 10 | | | | |
| 2a: Hinge | 2–4 x 10 | | | | |
| 2b: Push | 2–4 x 10 | | | | |
| *Intervals* | | | | | |
| | 3–6 x 30 seconds rest/ 60 seconds recovery | | | | |

| Workout B | | | | | |
| --- | --- | --- | --- | --- | --- |
| Category/exercise | Sets/reps | Workout 1 | Workout 2 | Workout 3 | Workout 4 |
| *Core* | | | | | |
| Dynamic stability | 2 x 10 | | | | |
| *Power* | | | | | |
| | 2 x 5–8 | | | | |
| *Strength* | | | | | |
| 1a: Single-leg stance | 2–4 x 10 | | | | |
| 1b: Push | 2–4 x 10 | | | | |
| 2a: Squat | 2–4 x 10 | | | | |
| 2b: Pull | 2–4 x 10 | | | | |
| *Intervals* | | | | | |
| | 3–6 x 30 seconds rest/ 60 seconds recovery | | | | |

### SUPERCHARGE IT!

If you want a sense of how Alwyn's clients typically do this program, do a mobility exercise after 1b and 2b. So you would do 1a, and rest until you catch your breath. Then you'd do 1b, but instead of resting, do one of the RAMP exercises for a few reps to each side. Rest 30 seconds, and repeat. Then do the same for 2a and 2b.

The mobility exercise won't interfere with your recovery from the strength exercises, but it will increase the overall density of the workout—the total amount of training you can squeeze into your hour in the weight room. It burns a few extra calories and should improve your conditioning over time.

It doesn't have to be a mobility exercise; you can also choose a core exercise, if you think it addresses a weak link or problem area.

# BASIC TRAINING III

### Workout A

| Category/exercise | Sets/reps | Workout 1 | Workout 2 | Workout 3 | Workout 4 |
|---|---|---|---|---|---|
| *Core* | | | | | |
| Dynamic stability | 2–3 x 10 | | | | |
| *Power* | | | | | |
| | 2 x 5–8 | | | | |
| *Strength* | | | | | |
| 1a: Hinge | 2–3 x 12 | | | | |
| 1b: Push | 2–3 x 12 | | | | |
| 1c: Lunge | 2–3 x 12 | | | | |
| 2a: Pull | 2–3 x 12 | | | | |
| 2b: Combination | 2–3 x 12 | | | | |
| *Intervals* | | | | | |
| | 4–6 by 30 seconds work/30 seconds recovery | | | | |

### Workout B

| Category/exercise | Sets/reps | Workout 1 | Workout 2 | Workout 3 | Workout 4 |
|---|---|---|---|---|---|
| *Core* | | | | | |
| Dynamic stability | 2–3 x 10 | | | | |
| *Power* | | | | | |
| | 2 x 5–8 | | | | |
| *Strength* | | | | | |
| 1a: Squat | 2–3 x 12 | | | | |
| 1b: Pull | 2–3 x 12 | | | | |
| 1c: Single-leg stance | 2–3 x 12 | | | | |
| 2a: Push | 2–3 x 12 | | | | |
| 2b: Combination | 2–3 x 12 | | | | |
| *Intervals* | | | | | |
| | 4–6 by 30 seconds work/30 seconds recovery | | | | |

### SUPERCHARGE IT!

This is how you'd do these workouts at Results Fitness: Do 1a, 1b, and 1c *without rest in between*, then rest at least 60 seconds after 1c. Same with 2a and 2b. Brutal? Probably, but I wouldn't know; I don't have the sand to attempt it. This works best for those who work out at home or in private gyms. In a commercial gym it's hard to do even two exercises without resting, much less three.

# BASIC TRAINING IV

This program offers a new twist on metabolic training. Instead of doing intervals, you'll select three strength exercises and one locomotion exercise (you'll find the locomotion options in Chapter 16). You'll do each exercise for 15 to 20 seconds, rather than counting reps. This takes away the incentive to race through each one. The trick is to pick four exercises that you can perform for at least 15 seconds at a time. For many of us that means a very light deadlift variation in Workout A, and perhaps bodyweight squats in Workout B. Even guys who can knock out high-rep sets of standard push-ups might want to consider elevated push-ups for either A or B. It's also fine to do unilateral exercises and split the reps between limbs. So if you were doing single-arm rows for one of your pull exercises, you might do 10 seconds with each arm.

## Workout A

| Category/exercise | Sets/reps | Workout 1 | Workout 2 | Workout 3 | Workout 4 |
|---|---|---|---|---|---|
| *Core* | | | | | |
| Dynamic stability | 2 x 10 | | | | |
| *Combination* | | | | | |
| | 2 x 8–10 | | | | |
| *Strength* | | | | | |
| 1a: Hinge | 3–4 x 10 | | | | |
| 1b: Push | 3–4 x 10 | | | | |
| 2a: Single-leg stance | 3–4 x 10 | | | | |
| 2b: Pull | 3–4 x 10 | | | | |
| *Metabolic* | | | | | |
| 3a: Hinge | 1–2 x 15–20 seconds | | | | |
| 3b: Push | 1–2 x 15–20 seconds | | | | |
| 3c: Locomotion | 1–2 x 15–20 seconds | | | | |
| 3d: Pull | 1–2 x 15–20 seconds | | | | |

## Workout B

| Category/exercise | Sets/reps | Workout 1 | Workout 2 | Workout 3 | Workout 4 |
|---|---|---|---|---|---|
| *Core* | | | | | |
| Stability | 2 x 30 seconds | | | | |
| *Combination* | | | | | |
| | 2 x 8–10 | | | | |
| *Strength* | | | | | |
| 1a: Squat | 3–4 x 10 | | | | |
| 1b: Pull | 3–4 x 10 | | | | |
| 2a: Lunge | 3–4 x 10 | | | | |
| 2b: Push | 3–4 x 10 | | | | |
| *Metabolic* | | | | | |
| 3a: Squat | 1–2 x 15–20 seconds | | | | |
| 3b: Pull | 1–2 x 15–20 seconds | | | | |
| 3c: Locomotion | 1–2 x 15–20 seconds | | | | |
| 3d: Push | 1–2 x 15–20 seconds | | | | |

## SUPERCHARGE IT!

Not challenging enough? Alwyn and his trainers do 1a, 1b, 2a, and 2b as one giant set (1a, 1b, 1c, 1d). Do all four exercises without a break in between, rest 90 seconds, and repeat.

# 20

# Hypertrophy

Now WE INTRODUCE A NEW WRINKLE: undulating periodization. You're going to do every exercise in your program with three different systems of sets and reps. In Hypertrophy I you do these:

- 4 sets of 6
- 3 sets of 12
- 2 sets of 20

In Hypertrophy II you do sets of 4, 8, and 12 reps, followed by Hypertrophy III with sets of 5, 10, and 15. That creates a need for a new type of bookkeeping, which you'll see on the workout charts.

Many readers will at first be confused by the designations of "Weeks 1 and 4," "Weeks 2 and 5," and "Weeks 3 and 6." In this case, a week isn't actually a week. It's just two workouts, A and B. The first time you do A and B, that's Week 1. The second time you do them, that's Week 2. Here's how a schedule might look, assuming you work out on Monday, Wednesday, and Friday. I used an actual month—April 2013—because April 1 conveniently falls on a Monday.

|  | Monday | Tuesday | Wednesday | Thursday | Friday | Saturday | Sunday |
|---|---|---|---|---|---|---|---|
| **April 1–7** | Workout A<br>Week 1<br>(4 x 6) | off | Workout B<br>Week 1<br>(3 x 12) | off | Workout A<br>Week 2<br>(2 x 20) | off | off |
| **April 8–14** | Workout B<br>Week 2<br>(4 x 6) | off | Workout A<br>Week 3<br>(3 x 12) | off | Workout B<br>Week 3<br>(2 x 20) | off | off |
| **April 15–21** | Workout A<br>Week 4<br>(4 x 6) | off | Workout B<br>Week 4<br>(3 x 12) | off | Workout A<br>Week 5<br>(2 x 20) | off | off |
| **April 22–28** | Workout B<br>Week 5<br>(4 x 6) | off | Workout A<br>Week 6<br>(3 x 12) | off | Workout B<br>Week 6<br>(2 x 20) | off | off |

I know we're hitting you with a lot of things to keep track of. Before you can do a single push-up or squat, you have to take note of Hypertrophy I, Workout A, exercise 1a, week 1, workout 1. On the positive side, you don't have to choose new exercises for all these different rep ranges. (You may want to in some cases; I'll get to that shortly.)

Let's use a pushing exercise, the dumbbell bench press, as an example. Say you start out using 40 pounds for sets of 6 and 20 pounds for sets of 12. (I picked a number somewhere in between what men and women would actually use.) Suppose that you set out to close the gap between those two exercises, so that by the end of Hypertrophy III you can do 12 reps with the weight you initially used for 6.

Maybe the second time you do sets of 12, you bump the weights up from 20 to 25 pounds. Then you move on to Hypertrophy II, in which you do sets of 4, 8, and 12 reps. This time you do the sets of 12 with 30 pounds. And even that seems light, because now you're doing sets of 8 with 40 pounds. That's right: You started out using 40 pounds for 6 reps, and now you can handle them for 8 reps.

Now you move on to Hypertrophy III, where you're doing sets of 5, 10, and 15 reps. You push yourself to use 40 pounds for sets of 10, and on your final set of your final workout, you go all out, and you manage to get 12 reps with 40 pounds. In just three months of training, you've gone from using 40-pound dumbbells for 6 reps to using them for 12. In the process you've also increased your performance in every other rep range.

You can do that with almost any exercise, in any movement pattern, and turn Alwyn's Hypertrophy workouts into a game you play against yourself. Heck, you can even take the next step and create incentives: Each time you double your reps with a starting weight, buy yourself a new kettlebell. (Just make sure you get free shipping if you buy online. It adds up!)

Now we get to a question I had, and I think many of you will have. Should you use the same exercises for every rep range? Alwyn prefers that you do most of the time. But there are exceptions. Take the bench presses I just described. I didn't use them for sets of 15 or 20. Instead I went for a push-up variation that would crush me in that rep range (which, frankly, is almost any push-up variation these days). On pulling exercises, stronger readers might do chin-ups for the low-rep sets (4, 5, or 6 reps), and band-assisted chin-ups for moderate reps (8 or 10). But for 12, 15, or 20, it probably makes sense to try a different vertical pulling exercise, like the half-kneeling lat pull-downs on page 134. Do 12 or more reps with each arm and you have a pretty decent metabolic challenge along with some core stimulation, on top of the targeted work for the pulling muscles in your back and arms.

Also keep in mind that you have three months to sort through all this. You may decide to stick with the same exercises for low and moderate reps in all three Hypertrophy programs, and switch up for higher reps. Just make sure you don't switch them up mid-program. So if you start off using one exercise the first time you do 2 sets of 20 in Hypertrophy II, use the same one the second time. Otherwise, you don't know if you're improving your performance or just amusing yourself in an iron-filled playpen.

# HYPERTROPHY I

| Workout A | | | |
|---|---|---|---|
| Category/exercise | Sets/reps | Workout 1 | Workout 2 |
| *Core* | | | |
| Stability | 1–2 x 30 seconds | | |
| Dynamic Stability | 1–2 x 10 | | |
| *Strength* | | | |
| 1a: Single-leg stance<br>Weeks 1 and 4<br>Weeks 2 and 5<br>Weeks 3 and 6 | <br>4 x 6<br>2 x 20<br>3 x 12 | | |
| 1b: Push<br>Weeks 1 and 4<br>Weeks 2 and 5<br>Weeks 3 and 6 | <br>4 x 6<br>2 x 20<br>3 x 12 | | |
| 2a: Hinge<br>Weeks 1 and 4<br>Weeks 2 and 5<br>Weeks 3 and 6 | <br>4 x 6<br>2 x 20<br>3 x 12 | | |
| 2b: Pull<br>Weeks 1 and 4<br>Weeks 2 and 5<br>Weeks 3 and 6 | <br>4 x 6<br>2 x 20<br>3 x 12 | | |
| *Complex* | | | |
| 3 exercises | 3–4 x 8 | | |

| Workout B | | | |
|---|---|---|---|
| **Category/exercise** | **Sets/reps** | **Workout 1** | **Workout 2** |
| *Core* | | | |
| Stability | 1–2 x 30 seconds | | |
| Dynamic Stability | 1–2 x 10 | | |
| *Strength* | | | |
| 1a: Lunge<br>Weeks 1 and 4<br>Weeks 2 and 5<br>Weeks 3 and 6 | <br>3 x 12<br>4 x 6<br>2 x 20 | | |
| 1b: Push<br>Weeks 1 and 4<br>Weeks 2 and 5<br>Weeks 3 and 6 | <br>3 x 12<br>4 x 6<br>2 x 20 | | |
| 2a: Squat<br>Weeks 1 and 4<br>Weeks 2 and 5<br>Weeks 3 and 6 | <br>3 x 12<br>4 x 6<br>2 x 20 | | |
| 2b: Pull<br>Weeks 1 and 4<br>Weeks 2 and 5<br>Weeks 3 and 6 | <br>3 x 12<br>4 x 6<br>2 x 20 | | |
| *Complex* | | | |
| 3 exercises | 3–4 x 8 | | |

# HYPERTROPHY II

| Workout A | | | |
|---|---|---|---|
| Category/exercise | Sets/reps | Workout 1 | Workout 2 |
| *Core* | | | |
| Stability | 1–2 x 30 seconds | | |
| Dynamic Stability | 1–2 x 10 | | |
| *Strength* | | | |
| 1a: Squat<br>Weeks 1 and 4<br>Weeks 2 and 5<br>Weeks 3 and 6 | <br>4 x 4<br>2 x 12<br>3 x 8 | | |
| 1b: Pull<br>Weeks 1 and 4<br>Weeks 2 and 5<br>Weeks 3 and 6 | <br>4 x 4<br>2 x 12<br>3 x 8 | | |
| 2a: Lunge<br>Weeks 1 and 4<br>Weeks 2 and 5<br>Weeks 3 and 6 | <br>4 x 4<br>2 x 12<br>3 x 8 | | |
| 2b: Push<br>Weeks 1 and 4<br>Weeks 2 and 5<br>Weeks 3 and 6 | <br>4 x 4<br>2 x 12<br>3 x 8 | | |
| *Complex* | | | |
| 3 exercises | 4–5 x 5 | | |

| Workout B | | | |
|---|---|---|---|
| **Category/exercise** | **Sets/reps** | **Workout 1** | **Workout 2** |
| *Core* | | | |
| Stability | 1–2 x 30 seconds | | |
| Dynamic Stability | 1–2 x 10 | | |
| *Strength* | | | |
| 1a: Hinge<br>Weeks 1 and 4<br>Weeks 2 and 5<br>Weeks 3 and 6 | <br>3 x 8<br>4 x 4<br>2 x 12 | | |
| 1b: Pull<br>Weeks 1 and 4<br>Weeks 2 and 5<br>Weeks 3 and 6 | <br>3 x 8<br>4 x 4<br>2 x 12 | | |
| 2a: Single-leg stance<br>Weeks 1 and 4<br>Weeks 2 and 5<br>Weeks 3 and 6 | <br>3 x 8<br>4 x 4<br>2 x 12 | | |
| 2b: Push<br>Weeks 1 and 4<br>Weeks 2 and 5<br>Weeks 3 and 6 | <br>3 x 8<br>4 x 4<br>2 x 12 | | |
| *Complex* | | | |
| 3 exercises | 4–5 x 5 | | |

# HYPERTROPHY III

| Workout A | | | |
|---|---|---|---|
| Category/exercise | Sets/reps | Workout 1 | Workout 2 |
| *Core* | | | |
| Dynamic Stability | 2 x 10 | | |
| *Strength* | | | |
| 1a: Lunge<br>Weeks 1 and 4<br>Weeks 2 and 5<br>Weeks 3 and 6 | <br>4 x 5<br>2 x 15<br>3 x 10 | | |
| 1b: Push<br>Weeks 1 and 4<br>Weeks 2 and 5<br>Weeks 3 and 6 | <br>4 x 5<br>2 x 15<br>3 x 10 | | |
| 2a: Hinge<br>Weeks 1 and 4<br>Weeks 2 and 5<br>Weeks 3 and 6 | <br>4 x 5<br>2 x 15<br>3 x 10 | | |
| 2b: Pull<br>Weeks 1 and 4<br>Weeks 2 and 5<br>Weeks 3 and 6 | <br>4 x 5<br>2 x 15<br>3 x 10 | | |
| *Complex* | | | |
| 3 exercises | 4–5 x 6 | | |

| Workout B | | | |
|---|---|---|---|
| Category/exercise | Sets/reps | Workout 1 | Workout 2 |
| *Core* | | | |
| Dynamic Stability | 2 x 10 | | |
| *Strength* | | | |
| 1a: Single-leg stance<br>Weeks 1 and 4<br>Weeks 2 and 5<br>Weeks 3 and 6 | 3 x 10<br>4 x 5<br>2 x 15 | | |
| 1b: Push<br>Weeks 1 and 4<br>Weeks 2 and 5<br>Weeks 3 and 6 | 3 x 10<br>4 x 5<br>2 x 15 | | |
| 2a: Squat<br>Weeks 1 and 4<br>Weeks 2 and 5<br>Weeks 3 and 6 | 3 x 10<br>4 x 5<br>2 x 15 | | |
| 2b: Pull<br>Weeks 1 and 4<br>Weeks 2 and 5<br>Weeks 3 and 6 | 3 x 10<br>4 x 5<br>2 x 15 | | |
| *Complex* | | | |
| 3 exercises | 4–5 x 6 | | |

# 21

# Strength & Power

THE THREE STRENGTH & POWER PROGRAMS are not only a big change from Basic Training and Hypertrophy, each of them is very different from the other two as well. I'll explain the specifics of each program when we get there. One key trait they all share: Your goal is to work with the heaviest possible load on the main exercise or exercises in each workout. That requires a warm-up strategy for each major lift.

As an example, let's look at Workout A in Strength & Power I. You see that you're alternating two exercises: hinge and push. Realistically, everybody's going to do a deadlift variation for the hinge, and a bench press or shoulder press for the push. The workout calls for 2 or 3 sets of 6 reps. Those are your work sets. You want to use your maximum weight—your 6-rep max, or 6RM—on each work set. To do that, you need to start with an educated guess of what your 6RM is. If you're doing the same exercises you used in Hypertrophy III, you have an easy choice. Just use the same weight you lifted for 4 sets of 5. If you're using different exercises, you'll have to make an educated guess.

Let's walk through the warm-up strategy for a fairly strong guy and a fairly strong woman, assuming both are using the same exercises: barbell deadlift and dumbbell bench press.

The guy plans to use 225 pounds for sets of 6 deadlifts, and 80-pound dumbbells for bench presses.

Since he's going to alternate the two exercises, he'll also alternate his warm-up sets. He starts with the bench press, doing 6 deliberately slow and easy reps with 40-pound dumbbells—half his work-set weight.

For the first deadlift warm-up, he'll use 135 pounds for 6 reps. There's nothing special about that number; it's just convenient because it allows him to start with a 45-pound plate on each side of the bar. His goal is to practice the lift, so he makes sure to put the bar down and reset his body on each repetition.

His next bench-press warm-up set is 4 or 5 reps with 60 pounds. He does these reps a little faster, as he would the work sets.

The second and final deadlift warm-up will probably be with 185 pounds. Again, it's just a convenient weight to use, since all he needs to do is slip a 25-pound plate on each side of the bar. This time he does 4 or 5 reps, again with the form he'll use for his work sets, resetting his body after each one.

Now he does one more warm-up set on the bench press, this time using 70-pound dumbbells for two or three reps. Why only two or three? The goal is to get your form right without wasting any energy you could use on your work sets. Why a third warm-up set for bench presses, but not deadlifts? Maybe it's just me, but after so many years in the gym I think lifts that stress the shoulders and knees require more practice and preparation. It's not that you don't need a full warm-up for hip-dominant lifts. But I think Alwyn's RAMP and core exercises do at least part of the job for you, especially when it comes to activating the muscles that stabilize your spine and pelvis.

A quick word about recovery between warm-up sets: When you're doing straight warm-up sets for a single exercise, you probably want at least 60 seconds in between, which may match the time it takes to change the weights. Take two minutes between your final warm-up and your first work set. You want to make sure the tank is full.

So now our guy is ready to start his work sets. Sure enough, he hits 6 reps with 225 pounds on the deadlift. It isn't exactly easy, but it doesn't feel like his best effort either. He decides he's going to use 245 for the next set.

The bench press is a different story. He only gets 5 reps with 80 pounds, and realizes he may have made two mistakes: First, he didn't rest a full two minutes after his set of deadlifts. Second, his final warm-up set with 70 pounds had felt heavier—that is, a bit more challenging—than he'd anticipated. He knows he should've listened to his body and done his work sets with 75 instead of 80 pounds.

After a full two minutes of rest, he gets all 6 reps with 245 on the deadlift. And after two more minutes of rest, he gets 6 reps with 75 pounds on the bench press. He uses those same weights for the third and final set of each exercise. He gets 6 reps on the deadlift, feeling even stronger on the third set. He only gets 4 on the bench press. The next time he does this workout, he plans to start heavier on the deadlift, going up to 255 pounds for his work sets. But on the bench press he's going to start lower, probably with 70 pounds. If that's too easy he'll go up to 75. He concedes that it'll take a while to reach 80.

The woman plans to use 135 pounds on the deadlift, and 40 pounds on the bench press. But she has a real challenge on the deadlift: No matter what she warms up with, the starting position for the bar will be lower than it will be for her work sets. The two best solutions are bumper plates (10- or 25-pound weight plates that are the same size as the 45s) or blocks (which would raise the bar a few inches above the floor), neither of which is available to her.

Her next-best choice is to do her warm-up sets in the squat rack, setting the side supports a few inches above the floor. For her first warm-up she uses just the 45-pound Olympic bar. For her second set she uses 95 pounds (the bar with a 25-pound plate on each side). Then she moves the barbell to the floor and loads it with a 45-pound plate on each side, giving her 135 pounds.

In between she does her bench press warm-ups, using 20 and 30 pounds. When 30 pounds feels heavier than expected, she decides to use 35 pounds for her work sets, instead of 40.

She gets only 5 reps on her first work set of deadlifts, leaving her with a tough choice: reduce the weight, or continue with fewer reps. She decides to continue with this weight, just because it would be such a pain to strip the bar and set up again in the rack. Besides, someone else is now using the rack for biceps curls, and she doesn't want to waste energy arguing. She struggles to get 5 reps on the second set, and gets only 4 on the third.

Meanwhile, 35-pound dumbbells on the bench press don't feel all that heavy. She gets 6 reps on the first two sets, and when she again gets 6 reps on the third set, she decides to keep going, knocking out 2 more reps for a total of 8.

Now she has her strategy in place for her next workout: She'll start with rack deadlifts using 115 pounds, with the goal of working up to 135 the following week.

But for bench presses, she's going to start with 40, with her eye on 45 or even 50 in the near future.

Two big points from these examples, which will come into play in every workout of every Strength & Power program:

1. Your warm-ups do more than prepare your muscles and joints for the lifts. They give you clues about what you can handle that day.
2. Rest periods can make or break your performance. Many of us are tempted to race through the warm-up sets to get to the heavy lifts. But if we don't fully recover during warm-ups, we're accumulating fatigue that will make our work sets less productive than they could be.

## STRENGTH & POWER I

As you know from my long (sorry, *really* long) introduction, your goal is to lift the most weight possible on the two exercises labeled "maximum strength & power": most likely deadlifts and bench presses in Workout A, and squats and chin-ups or rows in Workout B. That means thorough warm-ups, and full recovery between both warm-up and work sets.

Note that you're doing each workout six times in Strength & Power I. So you have time to get it right.

The next four exercises, however, are a different story. Labeled "muscle hypertrophy and endurance," your goal is the opposite. You want to accumulate fatigue. As you can see on the charts, the exercises are labeled 2a, 2b, 2c, and 2d, meaning you do them all consecutively, with about 60 seconds of rest after each. Then you repeat all four. If that's not possible in your gym, don't sweat it; you can alternate 2a and 2b, and then 2c and 2d, the way you have in all the previous programs. The point is to push yourself, to get exhausted and sweaty.

Your reward? Well, you get to pick any two exercises you want for Free Zone, as explained in Chapter 16, and do as many sets of 8 to 10 reps as you can in 5 minutes.

**Workout A**

| Category/exercise | Sets/reps | W1 | W2 | W3 | W4 | W5 | W6 |
|---|---|---|---|---|---|---|---|
| *Core* | | | | | | | |
| Stability | 2 x 30 seconds | | | | | | |
| Dynamic stability | 2 x 10 | | | | | | |
| *Maximum Strength & Power* | | | | | | | |
| 1a: Hinge | 2–3 x 6 | | | | | | |
| 1b: Push | 2–3 x 6 | | | | | | |
| *Muscle Hypertrophy & Endurance* | | | | | | | |
| 2a: Lunge | 2 x 15 | | | | | | |
| 2b: Pull | 2 x 15 | | | | | | |
| 2c: Single-leg stance | 2 x 15 | | | | | | |
| 2d: Push | 2 x 15 | | | | | | |
| *Free Zone* | | | | | | | |
| 2 exercises | 8–10 reps, as many sets as possible in 5 minutes | | | | | | |

**Workout B**

| Category/exercise | Sets/reps | W1 | W2 | W3 | W4 | W5 | W6 |
|---|---|---|---|---|---|---|---|
| *Core* | | | | | | | |
| Stability | 2 x 30 seconds | | | | | | |
| Dynamic stability | 2 x 10 | | | | | | |
| *Maximum Strength & Power* | | | | | | | |
| 1a: Squat | 2–3 x 6 | | | | | | |
| 1b: Pull | 2–3 x 6 | | | | | | |
| *Muscle Hypertrophy & Endurance* | | | | | | | |
| 2a: Single-leg stance | 2 x 15 | | | | | | |
| 2b: Push | 2 x 15 | | | | | | |
| 2c: Lunge | 2 x 15 | | | | | | |
| 2d: Pull | 2 x 15 | | | | | | |
| *Free Zone* | | | | | | | |
| 2 exercises | 8–10 reps, as many sets as possible in 5 minutes | | | | | | |

# STRENGTH & POWER II

Now we shift to four workouts—A, B, C, and D—each of which features one max-strength lift: squat, deadlift, and bench or shoulder press. (There's a different system for the pulling exercise, which I'll explain in a moment.) For that lift you'll do sets of 5, 5, 5, 5, and 8 reps. Use the heaviest weight possible for each of those sets, even if you have to drop the weight after the first or second set.

The final set of 8 is pure guts. You want to use about 90 percent of your 5-rep max—a weight that you lifted five times, but just barely. If it was 100 pounds, try to get 8 reps with 90. If it was 200 pounds, try for 180. Rest at least 2 minutes, and maybe even 3 or 4 minutes, before you attempt it.

You'll do each of these workouts three times, with a goal of increasing both your 5-rep max and the amount you use on that final set of 8.

For the pull in Workout B, you'll use the same technique as Strength & Power I: You're going for maximum performance in three consecutive sets. The difference is that you have a range of 3 to 6 reps. This covers the broadest spectrum of readers. For many, three chin-ups with your body weight is a max-effort set, while the strongest lifters may do weighted chin-ups for sets of 6. If you can't do at least three chin-ups, I recommend either band-assisted chin-ups (shown on page 145) or three-point dumbbell rows (page 136). If you do rows, shoot for sets of 5 or 6 with the heaviest possible weight. And of course do all the reps with each arm.

The rest of the workout is more conventional, although Alwyn gives you some twists. You'll notice that the exercises are the same in workouts A and C, and in B and D. You still want to improve your performance in those exercises, but your focus isn't on the weight you lift so much as the feel of the lifts. Choose exercises that are easy on your shoulders, knees, and lower back, and do the repetitions at a moderate pace that keeps your muscles under tension. Rest about 60 seconds after each set of each exercise.

You'll finish up, as before, with your choice of Free Zone exercises.

**Workout A**

| Category/exercise | Sets | Reps | Workout 1 | Workout 2 | Workout 3 |
|---|---|---|---|---|---|
| *Core* | | | | | |
| Dynamic stability | 2 | 10 | | | |
| *Maximum Strength & Power* | | | | | |
| 1: Squat | 5 | Set 1: 5<br>Set 2: 5<br>Set 3: 5<br>Set 4: 5<br>Set 5: 8 | | | |
| *Muscle Hypertrophy* | | | | | |
| 2a: Push | 2–3 | 8 | | | |
| 2b: Single-leg stance | 2–3 | 8 | | | |
| 3a: Pull | 3 | 8 | | | |
| 3b: Locomotion | 2 | 20–30 seconds | | | |
| *Free Zone* | | | | | |
| 2 exercises | 8–10 | As many as possible in 5 minutes | | | |

**Workout B**

| Category/exercise | Sets | Reps | Workout 1 | Workout 2 | Workout 3 |
|---|---|---|---|---|---|
| *Core* | | | | | |
| Dynamic stability | 2 | 10 | | | |
| *Maximum Strength & Power* | | | | | |
| 1: Pull | 3 | 3–6 | | | |
| *Muscle Hypertrophy* | | | | | |
| 2a: Lunge | 3 | 8 | | | |
| 2b: Push | 3 | 8 | | | |
| 3a: Pull | 2–3 | 12 | | | |
| 3b: Hinge | 2–3 | 8 | | | |
| *Free Zone* | | | | | |
| 2 exercises | 8–10 | As many as possible in 5 minutes | | | |

| Workout C | | | | | |
| --- | --- | --- | --- | --- | --- |
| Category/exercise | Sets | Reps | Workout 1 | Workout 2 | Workout 3 |
| *Core* | | | | | |
| Dynamic stability | 2 | 10 | | | |
| *Maximum Strength & Power* | | | | | |
| 1: Hinge | 5 | Set 1: 5<br>Set 2: 5<br>Set 3: 5<br>Set 4: 5<br>Set 5: 8 | | | |
| *Muscle Hypertrophy* | | | | | |
| 2a: Push | 2–3 | 8 | | | |
| 2b: Single-leg stance | 2–3 | 8 | | | |
| 3a: Pull | 3 | 8 | | | |
| 3b: Locomotion | 2 | 20–30 seconds | | | |
| *Free Zone* | | | | | |
| 2 exercises | 8–10 | As many as possible in 5 minutes | | | |

| Workout D | | | | | |
|---|---|---|---|---|---|
| Category/exercise | Sets | Reps | Workout 1 | Workout 2 | Workout 3 |
| *Core* | | | | | |
| Dynamic stability | 2 | 10 | | | |
| *Maximum Strength & Power* | | | | | |
| 1: Push | 5 | Set 1: 5<br>Set 2: 5<br>Set 3: 5<br>Set 4: 5<br>Set 5: 8 | | | |
| *Muscle Hypertrophy* | | | | | |
| 2a: Lunge | 3 | 8 | | | |
| 2b: Push | 3 | 8 | | | |
| 3a: Pull | 2–3 | 12 | | | |
| 3b: Hinge | 2–3 | 8 | | | |
| *Free Zone* | | | | | |
| 2 exercises | 8–10 | As many as possible in 5 minutes | | | |

# STRENGTH & POWER III

The structure is the same as Strength & Power II, but this time you'll use a technique called wave loading for your max-strength exercise. It's a neural trick to make heavy weights seem a bit lighter, and allow you to lift a little more than you otherwise would. It works like this:

Your first time through the workouts, you'll do two waves: 7 reps on your first set, 5 on the second, 3 on the third. Then you repeat the wave—sets of 7, 5, and 3 reps—only with heavier weights. The waves change in subsequent workouts, but they work the exact same way.

Let's walk through it, using any exercise you can imagine with the following weights.

Say you start with 50 pounds for 7 reps. Then you use 60 pounds for 5 reps, and 70 pounds for 3 reps. All three sets should feel challenging, but not like maximum efforts. For your second wave, you start with 55 pounds for 7 reps. After doing a set with 70, 55 doesn't feel heavier than 50 did. You follow that with 65 for 5 reps, and 75 for 3. It probably won't be until the final set that the weights on the second wave feel noticeably heavier.

After you do the 7-5-3 waves for all four workouts (A, B, C, and D), you do waves of 6, 4, and 2 reps, followed by waves of 5, 3, and 1 in your final workouts of this program. The weights get progressively heavier, workout by workout and wave by wave. By the end you should be close to a true one-rep max on three major lifts: squat, deadlift, and bench or shoulder press.

Rachel Cosgrove used this program to prepare for a powerlifting contest in which she not only won her division, she set a new deadlift record for the organization sanctioning the competition.

As before, you'll use a different technique for the pulling exercise. This time you'll do sets of 5 to 10 reps. The ideal strategy is to take the exercise you used for Strength & Power II, with the same weights (even if it's your body weight on chin-ups), and try to increase your reps.

**Workout A**

| Category/exercise | Sets | Reps | Workout 1 | Workout 2 | Workout 3 |
|---|---|---|---|---|---|
| *Core* | | | | | |
| Dynamic stability | 2 | 10 | | | |
| *Maximum Strength & Power* | | | | | |
| 1: Hinge | 5 | Wave | Set 1: 7<br>Set 2: 5<br>Set 3: 3<br>Set 4: 7<br>Set 5: 5<br>Set 6: 3 | Set 1: 6<br>Set 2: 4<br>Set 3: 2<br>Set 4: 6<br>Set 5: 4<br>Set 6: 2 | Set 1: 5<br>Set 2: 3<br>Set 3: 1<br>Set 4: 5<br>Set 5: 3<br>Set 6: 1 |
| *Muscle Hypertrophy* | | | | | |
| 2a: Pull | 2–3 | 10 | | | |
| 2b: Lunge | 2–3 | 10 | | | |
| 3a: Push | 2–3 | 12 | | | |
| 3b: Mobility | 2 | 10–12 | | | |
| *Free Zone* | | | | | |
| 2 exercises | 8–10 | As many as possible in 5 minutes | | | |

**Workout B**

| Category/exercise | Sets | Reps | Workout 1 | Workout 2 | Workout 3 |
|---|---|---|---|---|---|
| *Core* | | | | | |
| Dynamic stability | 2 | 10 | | | |
| *Maximum Strength & Power* | | | | | |
| 1: Push | 5 | Wave | Set 1: 7<br>Set 2: 5<br>Set 3: 3<br>Set 4: 7<br>Set 5: 5<br>Set 6: 3 | Set 1: 6<br>Set 2: 4<br>Set 3: 2<br>Set 4: 6<br>Set 5: 4<br>Set 6: 2 | Set 1: 5<br>Set 2: 3<br>Set 3: 1<br>Set 4: 5<br>Set 5: 3<br>Set 6: 1 |
| *Muscle Hypertrophy* | | | | | |
| 2a: Single-leg stance | 3 | 10 | | | |
| 2b: Pull | 3 | 10 | | | |
| 3a: Hinge | 3 | 10 | | | |
| 3b: Push | 3 | 10 | | | |
| *Free Zone* | | | | | |
| 2 exercises | 8–10 | As many as possible in 5 minutes | | | |

## Workout C

| Category/exercise | Sets | Reps | Workout 1 | Workout 2 | Workout 3 |
|---|---|---|---|---|---|
| *Core* | | | | | |
| Dynamic stability | 2 | 10 | | | |
| *Maximum Strength & Power* | | | | | |
| 1: Squat | 5 | Wave | Set 1: 7<br>Set 2: 5<br>Set 3: 3<br>Set 4: 7<br>Set 5: 5<br>Set 6: 3 | Set 1: 6<br>Set 2: 4<br>Set 3: 2<br>Set 4: 6<br>Set 5: 4<br>Set 6: 2 | Set 1: 5<br>Set 2: 3<br>Set 3: 1<br>Set 4: 5<br>Set 5: 3<br>Set 6: 1 |
| *Muscle Hypertrophy* | | | | | |
| 2a: Pull | 2–3 | 10 | | | |
| 2b: Lunge | 2–3 | 10 | | | |
| 3a: Push | 2–3 | 12 | | | |
| 3b: Mobility | 2 | 10–12 | | | |
| *Free Zone* | | | | | |
| 2 exercises | 8–10 | As many as possible in 5 minutes | | | |

## Workout D

| Category/exercise | Sets | Reps | Workout 1 | Workout 2 | Workout 3 |
|---|---|---|---|---|---|
| *Core* | | | | | |
| Dynamic stability | 2 | 10 | | | |
| *Maximum Strength & Power* | | | | | |
| 1: Pull | 3 | 5–10 | | | |
| *Muscle Hypertrophy* | | | | | |
| 2a: Single-leg stance | 3 | 10 | | | |
| 2b: Pull | 3 | 10 | | | |
| 3a: Hinge | 3 | 10 | | | |
| 3b: Push | 3 | 10 | | | |
| *Free Zone* | | | | | |
| 2 exercises | 8–10 | As many as possible in 5 minutes | | | |

# 22

# Sample Workouts

## BASIC TRAINING

I filled out the templates for all four Basic Training programs to show how the progression can work for someone who's healthy, relatively fit, has some experience in the weight room, and has no injuries that would affect exercise selection. These exercises should be appropriate for both genders and all ages. You'll see that I begin Basic Training I with "plank," "side plank," and "push-up" in the appropriate categories, and then in subsequent programs I use "plank variations," "side plank variations," and "push-up variations." In all three categories, I assume that you train with the most advanced variations you can use. (This will also come into play with "reverse lunge variations" a bit later.)

Three other assumptions:

- The Level 1 exercises are appropriately challenging for you in most categories.
- You can do at least 15 body-weight squats, which is why I start you off with the goblet squat, the Level 2 exercise.

- You have access to all the basic workout equipment (barbell, dumbbells, cable or bands, Swiss ball, a kettlebell or two, bench, and steps or boxes). If you don't have that equipment, just pick another exercise in the category.
- I don't select interval-training exercises for the first three programs. It really depends on (a) what you can do; (b) what you want to do; (c) what equipment you have available.

I could give you detailed notes on why I selected each exercise in each category, but it would put 99 percent of you to sleep, and this is already the longest book in the series. In general, I tried to avoid exercises that would put the same type of stress on knee or shoulder joints in the same workout. I also tried to consider the overall difficulty of the program. When I made an aggressive choice in one category, I tried to balance it with a less advanced exercise in another. This is especially important in the Metabolic Training section of Basic Training IV.

But I didn't take practicality into account. If you see combinations of exercises that you can't do in your health club or home gym, due to crowding or equipment limitations, just choose something else that works better for you.

## BASIC TRAINING I

| Workout A | | | | | |
|---|---|---|---|---|---|
| *Core* | | | | | |
| Stability: plank | 1–2 x 30 seconds | | | | |
| Dynamic Stability: side plank and row | 1–2 x 10* | | | | |
| *Power* | | | | | |
| Box jump | 2 x 5 | | | | |
| *Strength* | | | | | |
| 1a: Squat: Goblet squat | 1–2 x 15 | | | | |
| 1b: Pull: Standing cable row | 1–2 x 15* | | | | |
| 2a: Single-leg stance: Step-up | 1–2 x 15* | | | | |
| 2b: Push: Push-up | 1–2 x 15 | | | | |
| *Each side | | | | | |

**Workout B**

| Category/exercise | Sets/reps | Workout 1 | Workout 2 | Workout 3 | Workout 4 |
|---|---|---|---|---|---|
| *Core* | | | | | |
| Stability: Side plank | 1–2 x 30 seconds* | | | | |
| Dynamic stability: Plank with pulldown | 2 x 10* | | | | |
| *Combination* | | | | | |
| Reverse lunge and shoulder press | 2 x 5–8* | | | | |
| *Strength* | | | | | |
| 1a: Hinge: Swiss-ball supine hip extension | 1–2 x 15 | | | | |
| 1b: Push: Jackknife push-up | 1–2 x 15 | | | | |
| 2a: Lunge: Split squat | 1–2 x 15* | | | | |
| 2b: Pull: Kneeling lat pulldown | 1–2 x 15 | | | | |
| *Each side | | | | | |

# BASIC TRAINING II

**Workout A**

| Category/exercise | Sets/reps | Workout 1 | Workout 2 | Workout 3 | Workout 4 |
|---|---|---|---|---|---|
| *Core* | | | | | |
| Stability: Cable tall kneeling static hold | 2 x 30 seconds | | | | |
| *Combination* | | | | | |
| Romanian deadlift and row | 2 x 10 | | | | |
| *Strength* | | | | | |
| 1a: Lunge: Reverse lunge | 2–4 x 10* | | | | |
| 1b: Pull: Split-stance cable row | 2–4 x 10* | | | | |
| 2a: Hinge: Swiss-ball supine hip extension and leg curl | 2–4 x 10 | | | | |
| 2b: Push: Push-up variations | 2–4 x 10 | | | | |
| *Each side | | | | | |

**Workout B**

| Category/exercise | Sets/reps | Workout 1 | Workout 2 | Workout 3 | Workout 4 |
|---|---|---|---|---|---|
| *Core* | | | | | |
| Dynamic stability: Push-away | 2 x 10 | | | | |
| *Power* | | | | | |
| Jump squat | 2 x 5–8 | | | | |
| *Strength* | | | | | |
| 1a: Single-leg stance: Offset-loaded step-up | 2–4 x 10* | | | | |
| 1b: Push: Jackknife push-up with elevated feet | 2–4 x 10 | | | | |
| 2a: Squat: Front squat | 2–4 x 10 | | | | |
| 2b: Pull: Single-arm half-kneeling lat pulldown | 2–4 x 10* | | | | |
| *Each side | | | | | |

# BASIC TRAINING III

**Workout A**

| Category/exercise | Sets/reps | Workout 1 | Workout 2 | Workout 3 | Workout 4 |
|---|---|---|---|---|---|
| *Core* | | | | | |
| Dynamic stability: Mountain climber | 2–3 x 10* | | | | |
| *Power* | | | | | |
| Kettlebell swing† | 2 x 5–8 | | | | |
| *Strength* | | | | | |
| 1a: Hinge: Romanian deadlift | 2–3 x 12 | | | | |
| 1b: Push: Push-up variations | 2–3 x 12 | | | | |
| 1c: Lunge: Reverse lunge variations | 2–3 x 12* | | | | |
| 2a: Pull: Dumbbell two-point row | 2–3 x 12* | | | | |
| 2b: Combination: Squat and press | 2–3 x 12 | | | | |
| *Each side | | | | | |
| †No kettlebell? Continue with jump squats. | | | | | |

| Workout B | | | | | |
|---|---|---|---|---|---|
| Category/exercise | Sets/reps | Workout 1 | Workout 2 | Workout 3 | Workout 4 |
| *Core* | | | | | |
| Dynamic stability: Cable tall kneeling chop | 2–3 x 10* | | | | |
| *Power* | | | | | |
| Explosive push-up | 2 x 5–8 | | | | |
| *Strength* | | | | | |
| 1a: Squat: Offset overhead squat | 2–3 x 12 | | | | |
| 1b: Pull: Standing lat pulldown | 2–3 x 12 | | | | |
| 1c: Single-leg stance: Single-leg Romanian deadlift | 2–3 x 12* | | | | |
| 2a: Push: Dumbbell shoulder press | 2–3 x 12 | | | | |
| 2b: Combination: Push-up and one-arm row | 2–3 x 12* | | | | |
| *Each side | | | | | |

# BASIC TRAINING IV

| Workout A | | | | | |
|---|---|---|---|---|---|
| Category/exercise | Sets/reps | Workout 1 | Workout 2 | Workout 3 | Workout 4 |
| *Core* | | | | | |
| Dynamic stability: Swiss-ball rollout | 2 x 10 | | | | |
| *Combination* | | | | | |
| Squat and press | 2 x 8–10 | | | | |
| *Strength* | | | | | |
| 1a: Hinge: Rack deadlift | 3–4 x 10 | | | | |
| 1b: Push: Standing single-arm cable chest press | 3–4 x 10* | | | | |
| 2a: Single-leg stance: Step-up *(any variation)* | 3–4 x 10* | | | | |
| 2b: Pull: Inverted row | 3–4 x 10 | | | | |
| *Metabolic* | | | | | |
| 3a: Hinge: Romanian deadlift | 1–2 x 15–20 seconds | | | | |
| 3b: Push: Push-up variations | 1–2 x 15–20 seconds | | | | |
| 3c: Locomotion: Any loaded carry in Chapter 16 | 1–2 x 15–20 seconds | | | | |
| 3d: Pull: Standing cable row | 1–2 x 15–20 seconds | | | | |
| *Each side | | | | | |

| Workout B | | | | | |
| Category/exercise | Sets/reps | Workout 1 | Workout 2 | Workout 3 | Workout 4 |
| --- | --- | --- | --- | --- | --- |
| *Core* | | | | | |
| Stability: Side plank variations | 2 x 30 seconds* | | | | |
| *Combination* | | | | | |
| Romanian deadlift and row | 2 x 8–10 | | | | |
| *Strength* | | | | | |
| 1a: Squat: Front squat | 3–4 x 10 | | | | |
| 1b: Pull: Dumbbell three-point row | 3–4 x 10* | | | | |
| 2a: Lunge: Split squat, rear foot elevated | 3–4 x 10* | | | | |
| 2b: Push: Dumbbell bench press | 3–4 x 10 | | | | |
| *Metabolic* | | | | | |
| 3a: Squat: Goblet squat | 1–2 x 15–20 seconds | | | | |
| 3b: Pull: Kneeling lat pulldown | 1–2 x 15–20 seconds | | | | |
| 3c: Locomotion: Bear crawl | 1–2 x 15–20 seconds | | | | |
| 3d: Push: Dumbbell shoulder press | 1–2 x 15–20 seconds | | | | |
| *Each side | | | | | |

## HYPERTROPHY

Rather than fill in the templates for all three programs, I started and stopped with Hypertrophy I. By the time you're ready for Hypertrophy II and III, you should understand Alwyn's system (not to mention your own body) well enough to pick exercises. As a secondary goal, I wanted to show a progression from Basic Training IV to Hypertrophy I.

I leave the complexes up to you. The key to selecting the best combination of exercises is to take into account what you've already done in the workout. If your complex includes shoulder presses, for example, and you've already done shoulder presses for your push exercise, you're going to have some very tired shoulders and triceps. There's nothing wrong with giving those muscles a double-dose of growth stimuli; I just wanted to warn you that you may be in for a surprise. (I write this based on the very recent experience of having my shoulders poop out halfway through my second complex.)

# HYPERTROPHY I

| Workout A | | | |
|---|---|---|---|
| Category/exercise | Sets/reps | Workout 1 | Workout 2 |
| *Core* | | | |
| Stability: Plank variations | 1–2 x 30 seconds | | |
| Dynamic Stability: Cable half-kneeling chop | 1–2 x 10* | | |
| *Strength* | | | |
| 1a: Single-leg stance: Single-leg Romanian deadlift<br>Weeks 1 and 4<br>Weeks 2 and 5<br>Weeks 3 and 6 | <br>4 x 6*<br>2 x 20<br>3 x 12 | | |
| 1b: Push: Dumbbell bench press†<br>Weeks 1 and 4<br>Weeks 2 and 5<br>Weeks 3 and 6 | <br>4 x 6<br>2 x 20<br>3 x 12 | | |
| 2a: Hinge: Deadlift†<br>Weeks 1 and 4<br>Weeks 2 and 5<br>Weeks 3 and 6 | <br>4 x 6<br>2 x 20<br>3 x 12 | | |
| 2b: Pull: Dumbbell three-point row†<br>Weeks 1 and 4<br>Weeks 2 and 5<br>Weeks 3 and 6 | <br>4 x 6*<br>2 x 20<br>3 x 12 | | |
| *Each side | | | |
| †You can substitute another exercise for the 20-rep sets (push-ups, Swiss-ball hip extensions/leg curls, and standing cable rows, for example). | | | |

| Workout B | | | |
| --- | --- | --- | --- |
| Category/exercise | Sets/reps | Workout 1 | Workout 2 |
| *Core* | | | |
| Stability: Side-plank variations | 1–2 x 30 seconds* | | |
| Dynamic Stability: Swiss-ball mountain climber | 1–2 x 10* | | |
| *Strength* | | | |
| 1a: Lunge: Bulgarian split squat | | | |
| Weeks 1 and 4 | 3 x 12* | | |
| Weeks 2 and 5 | 4 x 6 | | |
| Weeks 3 and 6 | 2 x 20 | | |
| 1b: Push: Dumbbell shoulder press† | | | |
| Weeks 1 and 4 | 3 x 12 | | |
| Weeks 2 and 5 | 4 x 6 | | |
| Weeks 3 and 6 | 2 x 20 | | |
| 2a: Squat: Front squat† | | | |
| Weeks 1 and 4 | 3 x 12 | | |
| Weeks 2 and 5 | 4 x 6 | | |
| Weeks 3 and 6 | 2 x 20 | | |
| 2b: Pull: Inverted row† | | | |
| Weeks 1 and 4 | 3 x 12 | | |
| Weeks 2 and 5 | 4 x 6 | | |
| Weeks 3 and 6 | 2 x 20 | | |

*Each side

†Substitutions for 20-rep sets might include jackknife push-ups, goblet or Zercher squats, and half-kneeling lat pull-downs.

## STRENGTH & POWER

Again, I'll show you a sample of Strength & Power I, and turn you loose on the final two programs. Remember that you also get to choose Free Zone exercises for these workouts.

# STRENGTH & POWER I

| Workout A | | | | | | | |
|---|---|---|---|---|---|---|---|
| Category/exercise | Sets/reps | Workout 1 | Workout 2 | Workout 3 | Workout 4 | Workout 5 | Workout 6 |
| *Core* | | | | | | | |
| Stability: Plank variations | 2 x 30 seconds | | | | | | |
| Dynamic stability: Swiss-ball jackknife | 2 x 10 | | | | | | |
| *Maximum Strength & Power* | | | | | | | |
| 1a: Hinge: Deadlift | 2–3 x 6 | | | | | | |
| 1b: Push: Dumbbell bench press | 2–3 x 6 | | | | | | |
| *Muscle Hypertrophy & Endurance* | | | | | | | |
| 2a: Lunge: Forward lunge | 2 x 15* | | | | | | |
| 2b: Pull: Standing lat pulldown | 2 x 15 | | | | | | |
| 2c: Single-leg stance: Overhead step-up | 2 x 15* | | | | | | |
| 2d: Push: Modified handstand push-up | 2 x 15 | | | | | | |
| *Each side | | | | | | | |

**Workout B**

| Category/exercise | Sets/reps | Workout 1 | Workout 2 | Workout 3 | Workout 4 | Workout 5 | Workout 6 |
|---|---|---|---|---|---|---|---|
| *Core* | | | | | | | |
| Stability: Side-plank variations | 2 x 30 seconds* | | | | | | |
| Dynamic stability: Suspended fallout | 2 x 10 | | | | | | |
| *Maximum Strength & Power* | | | | | | | |
| 1a: Squat: Front squat | 2–3 x 6 | | | | | | |
| 1b: Pull: Chin-up | 2–3 x 6 | | | | | | |
| *Muscle Hypertrophy & Endurance* | | | | | | | |
| 2a: Single-leg stance: Single-leg Romanian deadlift | 2 x 15* | | | | | | |
| 2b: Push: Dumbbell shoulder press | 2 x 15 | | | | | | |
| 2c: Lunge: Reverse lunge variations | 2 x 15* | | | | | | |
| 2d: Pull: Dumbbell three-point row | 2 x 15* | | | | | | |
| *Each side | | | | | | | |

# PART 5

# THE POSTGAME

# 23

# You Know You Want to Ask

THIS IS THE FIFTH BOOK IN the New Rules of Lifting series. We can never anticipate all the questions that arise, but there are patterns that emerge with each one. Before you ask anything, I recommend these resources:

- *The New Rules of Lifting Supercharged.* Believe it or not, it helps to read the book before asking questions about it.
- The NROL forums at jpfitness.com. Your questions are typically answered within a day—and sometimes within an hour or two—by someone who's read the book and done the programs.
- On Facebook, I try to answer questions on the New Rules of Lifting page when they come up, and Alwyn does speed coaching on his fan page (facebook.com/ AlwynCosgroveFanPage) when he gets a chance. You know the drill: "like" both pages, follow us on Twitter, subscribe to our newsletters, collect our commemorative bobbleheads . . .
- I also recommend downloading the free training logs at werkit.com, designed by Aoife Hammersmith. They're a great way to track and organize your workouts,

and they're pretty much essential if you bought *Supercharged* for your Kindle and have trouble reading the workout charts.

Now let's look at some of the questions that come up most often:

### "What *is* all this? I mean, what the hell?"

I see your point. It's certainly easier to show people exactly what to do and take away the burden of choice. But we did that in the first three books, and most of the questions that arose concerned exercise substitutions. "Can I do *this* instead of *that*?" For our fourth book, *NROL for Life*, we decided to put those decisions in the readers' hands. Now with *Supercharged* we're doing that again, only with more programs and thus more exercise choices.

Your workouts, however, don't have to be complicated. Let's walk through the system:

- You have ten programs—four in Basic Training, three in Hypertrophy, three in Strength & Power. But you only do one at a time. Almost everyone will start at the beginning, with Basic Training I.
- Before you start, you need to select exercises for two workouts: A and B. All you have to worry about for the next four weeks is improving your performance on those exercises in those workouts.
- If you outgrow an exercise in the middle of a program—you've hit the maximum time or number of repetitions—then you'll want to move up to the next exercise in that category. This will happen for most readers on core exercises and for many on push-up variations. Otherwise, you can just keep going until you get to the next program.
- When you finish a program, select exercises for the next program. Most of the time you'll want to move up to slightly more advanced variations. If you started at Level 1, move up to Level 2. Or you can try the "Supercharge it!" options. Do those for the next four weeks. Continue like that into infinity.

### "Can I do the same exercises for multiple programs?"

Sure, if it's a key exercise and your performance is improving from workout to workout. Particularly in Strength & Power most of us will end up settling on one key exercise variation for each of the four major movement patterns: squat, deadlift, push (bench press or shoulder press), and pull (row or chin-up).

I encourage you to mix and match lunge, single-leg-stance, and core variations from program to program, along with whatever you decide to do for metabolic training. Not only is it more fun to train that way, it gives your joints some relief, and your muscles some new challenges.

### "I can do just about every exercise in every category. How do I decide which ones to use?"

Three rules:

*For fat loss, choose the most difficult exercises to perform.* It probably doesn't matter if the difficulty comes from the number of moving parts, or the challenge of stabilizing nonmoving parts. If it makes you sweat, jacks up your heart rate, and requires some time to get your breathing back to normal, it's probably going to induce a level of metabolic stress that will burn more calories, both during and after the workout. For me, these are single-arm push and pull exercises with a balance component (like the half-kneeling single-arm lat pulldown shown on page 134), and the lower-body exercises with an offset load.

*For hypertrophy, choose the exercises that offer the most direct line of resistance.* Push-ups or dumbbell presses. Dumbbell rows. Romanian deadlifts. Front squats. The exercises are somewhat simple, and tend to work best with moderate to high repetitions, allowing you to produce a high level of fatigue in your biggest muscles. They also allow you to feel the targeted muscles in action.

*For strength and power, choose the exercises that allow you to lift the most weight from the most stable position.* Bench presses, chin-ups, deadlifts, and squats use the most muscle to push or pull the heaviest loads. They lend themselves to low-repetition sets in which each rep feels like something close to a maximum effort.

### "Can I exercise on the days in between NROL workouts?"

You can and probably should. The key is to choose activities that either help you recover from strength training, or don't affect it either way. Yoga, for example, can be a great exercise choice between strength workouts, assuming you either know what you're doing or take a class with an instructor who knows what he or she is doing. (People do get hurt practicing yoga with poor form.) If you're an advanced lifter whose body is conditioned to high levels of fatigue and metabolic stress, you have a pretty good idea of how much you can do between workouts. For everyone else, this big question breaks down into three different questions:

### "Can I do additional strength training?"

If you're talking about relatively high-rep, low-load exercises, sure. Alwyn works out almost every day. You could do supplemental workouts that include core and mobility training, body-weight exercises, routines that use a specialized type of equipment (TRX, kettlebells, sandbags . . .). The key is to avoid high levels of muscle fatigue and mechanical tension. That will affect your recovery and probably compromise your results.

### "Can I do high-intensity intervals?"

I would say this is a better option for highly trained athletes, and not the best choice for someone who has a lot of weight to lose or is looking to get back into shape after a long layoff. Intervals work by creating a high level of metabolic stress, and sometimes produce joint stress as well. Over time, too many high-effort workouts with too few breaks in between leave you mentally exhausted, along with the residual fatigue your body absorbs.

That said, heavier and less fit readers can get a lot out of low-intensity intervals. Jog for a minute, walk for two minutes. It doesn't have to be any more complicated or draining than that.

### "Can I do endurance training?"

Of course, if it's something you like to do, want to do, and/or need to do for your job or your sport. Alwyn's workouts—particularly the four Basic Training programs—are a terrific complement to endurance training. As I was writing *Supercharged* a radio host told me that the *NROL for Abs* workouts had transformed his running performance. By improving his strength, mobility, and core fitness he was able to run faster despite running fewer miles in training.

I'll just throw out the usual cautions:

As Alwyn has said in previous books, running is not an entry-level activity. It's a high-impact sport requiring a moderately high level of fitness before you begin piling up the miles.

Another concern is specialization. If your goal is to run marathons or compete in triathlons, you have to focus on those and train your body to become more efficient at running, riding, and/or swimming long distances. Strength training can be a useful adjunct, but if you try to focus on building strength and muscle mass while also improving endurance, you'll end up with disappointing results all around. It also works the other way. If your main goal is to get bigger and stronger, a serious endurance program will almost certainly limit your gains.

Choose one or the other as your main focus, and use the other as an adjunct. Sports have seasons; you can schedule your workouts the same way. Train primarily for endurance half the year, and primarily for strength and muscle mass the other half. It's never all or nothing. As any Star Wars geek can tell you, only a Sith deals in absolutes.

### "Can I repeat the programs?"

Absolutely. You could probably cycle through the four Basic Training programs two or three times before you stopped getting results. (Remember that Basic Training I, II, and III are very similar to the three programs in *NROL for Life,* so if you've done those a couple times already, you'll see diminishing returns by performing them more than once here.) The Hypertrophy programs should be worth a second time around if you like them and want to continue. And the Strength & Power programs have a built-in periodization element. Following Strength & Power III, you could use S&P I as a restorative program, to get your body re-energized for another run at S&P II and III.

### "No offense, but the nutrition info is kind of skimpy. What do I eat to get the results I want?"

None taken. This is primarily a training book, but of course you can't get all you want from your training without modifying your diet. You have to eat a decent amount of food both to perform Alwyn's workouts the way they're intended, and to recover from them. If I could come up with a nutrition program to match the depth and versatility of Alwyn's training programs, I'd gladly make that the next book. For now, here's a reasonable diet in bullet points:

- You can get bigger or leaner with two, three, five, or eight meals a day . . . as long as you're consistent in whatever you choose to do. This applies to people who use intermittent fasting as well. Jumping from one thing to another makes it hard to know what works and what doesn't.
- Most of us should aim for a relatively high-protein diet. This is especially important when you're cutting calories with the goal of losing fat. Alan Aragon suggests having 1 gram of protein per pound of target body weight per day, and that makes as much sense as anything I've heard or read.

- Most meals should have a base of protein, if for no other reason than because it's easier to eat a lot of protein when you spread it out across all your meals.

- Try to eat some protein an hour or two before working out, and then some more shortly after. Twenty grams of high-quality protein per meal seems to be enough for most of us, although more is fine. If you work out first thing in the morning on an empty stomach, you probably want a shake or protein-rich meal as soon as possible after you finish.

- Once your protein needs are met, you can do well with just about any mix of high-quality, unprocessed carbs and fats. If protein is 20 to 30 percent of your total calories, you could split the remaining 70 to 80 percent equally and probably do fine.

- What does that mean? Well, protein has 4 calories per gram. If your target weight is, say, 140 pounds, you're looking at 560 calories from protein, or about 25 percent of a 2,200-calorie-a-day diet.

- Is 2,200 calories a day a good target? I don't know. The best advice I can offer is to record three days' worth of meals and snacks on an online calculator like the ones at fitday.com, livestrong.com/thedailyplate, or sparkpeople.com. My friend Roland Denzel recommends the free Fitbit nutrition-tracking app for iPhone or Android, at fitbit.com. Be honest and make it three typical days, not three days of feeling like the nutrition police are watching you. See what you're eating now. Then figure out what you can cut if you want to lose weight, or what you can add if you need to gain.

- If you need to cut, start with processed foods. They typically offer the most calories with the least nutrition. Those with fat skew toward one type (omega-6 polyunsaturated fat, mostly from soybean oil) and one or two sources of carbohydrate (usually corn or wheat). Sometimes these foods are "fortified" with a bunch of the vitamins and minerals that were removed with processing, but that's just for marketing. The real goal is to engineer food to delay satiation so you eat more than you otherwise would. They get paid, and you get fat.

- If your goal is weight loss, you'll probably do best with fewer carbs than you're eating now. You'll need to replace some of them with protein and fat. Some of the best "diet" foods are the ones from animal sources—meat, fish, eggs, dairy—that contain a mix of high-quality protein and a range of saturated and unsaturated fats. Seek out some high-fat plant foods, like avocados and nuts, again for the variety of nutrients.

- If you're looking to add muscle, or fuel athletic performance with a heavy training schedule, carbs are your friend.

- Which carbs? Depends on which group of experts you listen to. Me, I go for fruit, vegetables, and nuts, with some legumes (beans, peas, lentils, peanuts) and the occasional potato or sweet potato. The less bread and pasta I have, the less I weigh. Rice has always seemed kind of ethereal to me. I don't eat much of it, but when I do, I don't notice it one way or the other. In my stomach it's like magician's flash paper—it's there, and then it's not. Figure out a mix that works with your metabolism and your preferences; I don't think anyone can do it for you.

- The great thing about fruit is that it exists to be shat. That's how it evolved to propagate itself. Animals eat it, enjoy the taste, use the carbohydrates for energy, and excrete the seeds. A perfect circle.

- In general, I'm not a big fan of obsessing over single nutrients. I don't take any vitamins, multi or singular. The one exception is fish oil. I don't have many sources of omega-3 polyunsaturated fats in my daily diet, so I supplement with a couple of pills a day.

## "Does strength training really have to be this complicated?"

No. You can do anything you download off the Internet for a few weeks and see results. You can find progressive programs that lay out everything for you. And those are fine. The first three books in the NROL series did exactly that, as have most of the workout books I've been involved with over the years. At some point, however, you have to learn to modify programs to accommodate your own injuries or limitations, and to address your imbalances and weak links. I know as well as anyone that if you start with a blank slate, you're going to fill it in with exercises that only play to your strengths or accommodate your limitations, while never addressing your weak links. I always do that eventually, and I assume you do too.

Alwyn wants to give you the best of both worlds: a workout template that doesn't allow you to avoid altogether the movements you don't like or that make you feel momentarily awkward, while at the same time giving you the ability to move forward at your own speed—to get as much done as you can or will within a reasonable framework.

There's an art and a science to training. Alwyn is in charge of the science. He's relentlessly analytical about how different components of his programs contribute to the overall effect. The basics of exercise science don't change, but the applications do.

Just in the time Alwyn has been training clients, which roughly overlaps with the time I've been writing about fitness, our emphasis has changed dramatically. We started out talking about muscles—lift like *this* to build *that*. Then we shifted the emphasis to joint actions. Then, as we launched the NROL series, we emphasized movement patterns. At the same time, we tried to answer the other questions that arose about the way we lift: What effect does load have? Do you have to lift heavy weights, relative to your maximum strength, or can you get similar results with lighter weights and a higher overall volume? What about lifting speed? Should you slow down? Speed up? What if you quit counting reps and time your sets instead?

But from the outside, a lot of what we do looks exactly like what we've always done. We're still doing squats, deadlifts, lunges, presses, rows, and chin-ups. We're reintroducing push-ups while de-emphasizing crunches and sit-ups. As our world forces us to sit for more hours each day, our workouts change to keep us on our feet, to do everything we can to counteract the fitness-sapping effects of our sedentary lives. And we end up with workouts that sometimes resemble the gym classes, football practices, or military training of days gone by. We even use terms like "boot camp" and "basic training" as selling points.

It constantly changes, and yet it's all the same.

What matters is what you do today, and tomorrow, and the days and weeks and months and years to come. If it makes sense, if it works, if it gives you the results you want from the effort you're willing to exert, then you've found something that eludes almost everyone who begins a fitness program.

Will the workouts in *Supercharged* give you those results? We think so, and we hope so. The important question is, will you make it so?

# Appendix: The Rules

These are the rules from all three *NROL* books, starting with the basic rules of exercise:

1. Do something.
2. Do something you like.
3. The rest is just details.

These are the original New Rules of Lifting:

1. The best muscle-building exercises are the ones that use your muscles the way they're designed to work.
2. Exercises that use lots of muscles in coordinated action are better than those that force muscles to work in isolation.
3. To build size, you must build strength.
4. To build size and strength, you must train hard but infrequently, with plenty of recovery time between workouts.
5. The goal of each workout is to set a record.

6. The weight you lift is a tool to reach your goals. It is not a goal by itself.
7. Don't "do the machines."
8. A workout is only as good as the adaptations it produces.
9. There is no magic system of exercises, sets, and reps.
10. Don't judge a system by the physique of the person promoting it.
11. You'll get better results working your ass off on a bad program than you will loafing through a good program.
12. Fast lifting is not more dangerous than slow lifting.
13. A good warm-up doesn't have to make your body warm.
14. Stretching is not a warm-up.
15. You don't need to warm up to stretch.
16. Lifting by itself may increase your flexibility.
17. Aerobic fitness is not a matter of life and death.
18. You don't need to do endurance exercise to burn fat.
19. When you combine serious strength training with serious endurance exercise, your body will probably choose endurance over muscle and strength.
20. If it's not fun, you're doing something wrong.

The New Rules of Lifting for Women:

1. The purpose of lifting weights is to build muscle.
2. Muscle is hard to build.
3. Results come from hard work.
4. Hard work includes lifting heavier weights.
5. From time to time, you have to break some of the old rules.
6. No workout will make you taller.
7. Muscles in men and women are essentially identical.
8. Muscle strength is a matter of life and death.
9. A muscle's "pump" is not the same as muscle growth.
10. Endurance exercise is an option, not a necessity, for fat loss.
11. "Aerobics" doesn't mean what you think it means.
12. Calorie restriction is the worst idea ever.
13. Traditional weight-loss advice is fatally flawed.
14. To reach your goals, you may need to eat more.
15. On balance, a balanced macro diet is best.
16. Protein is the queen of macronutrients.

**17.** More meals are better than fewer.

**18.** Don't do programs designed for someone else's needs.

**19.** You don't need to isolate small muscles to make them bigger and stronger.

**20.** Every exercise is a "core" exercise.

**21.** The biggest blocks to your success could be the ones you've erected.

The New Rules of Lifting for Abs:

**1.** The most important role of the abdominal muscles is to protect your spine.

**2.** You can't protect your spine by doing exercises that damage it.

**3.** The size of your abdominal muscles doesn't matter.

**4.** The appearance of your abs doesn't matter either.

**5.** The core includes all the muscles that attach to your hips, pelvis, and lower back.

**6.** The lats are part of the core.

**7.** The crunch is not a core exercise.

**8.** Your spine is already flexed, and flexing it more just makes it worse.

**9.** Stability in your lower back depends on mobility in the joints above and below it.

**10.** You can't out-exercise a hunger-inducing lifestyle.

**11.** Your computer is the enemy of your abs.

**12.** TV and video games are almost as bad as your computer.

**13.** You can sleep your way to a better body . . . or not sleep your way to a bigger belly.

**14.** "Convenience" food is designed to make you eat more convenience food.

**15.** Processed food makes you stupid and depressed.

**16.** All that said, calories still matter more than anything else.

**17.** Don't do a complicated intervention unless you've tried all the simple ones.

The New Rules of Lifting for Life:

**1.** The older you are, the more important it is to train.

**2.** The goal of training is to change something.

**3.** Your body won't change without consistent hard work.

**4.** Hard work doesn't mean beating the crap out of yourself every time you train.

**5.** You're not a kid anymore. Don't train like one.

**6.** Decline is inevitable.

**7.** How fast you decline is up to you.

**8.** You are not a rural Okinawan.

9. Everyone is injured. But not every injury hurts.
10. If an activity hurts, stop doing it.
11. If it hurts after you do it, it may or may not be a problem.
12. Never try to fix an acute injury by stretching it.
13. When in doubt, refer out.
14. Exercise burns calories. Sometimes that's a problem.
15. "Fat-burning" exercise doesn't always burn fat.
16. Alwyn figured this out a long time ago.
17. It's actually kind of hard to gain weight.
18. We don't really move less.
19. Tasty food makes it too easy to gain weight, and too hard to lose it.
20. Every pound you don't gain is one you don't have to worry about losing.
21. Self-control, like muscle strength, can improve with training.
22. Weight management has little to do with self-control.
23. A weight-loss plan is good for six months, max.
24. Weight maintenance requires new strategies and a different skill set.

Finally, The New Rules of Lifting Supercharged:

1. It's great to be good.
2. Once you're good, you need to get strong.
3. "Strong" is an aspiration, not an endpoint.
4. The only guaranteed way to get strong is with a focused, progressive program.
5. To stay strong, you must move well.
6. This means you.
7. A real lifter knows how to squat.
8. A well-trained butt is a thing of beauty.
9. Your lats are core muscles. Get off your rump and train them that way.
10. Nobody ever died of small pecs.
11. The lines between "strength," "cardio," and "flexibility" aren't as clear as you think.
12. The benefits of the program exceed the sum of the individual parts.
13. Power is to fitness as fitness is to health.
14. The muscle fairy has a sick sense of humor.
15. Every program is a hypertrophy program.
16. Every program is a strength program.
17. Every program is a fat-loss program.

**18.** Muscle building takes place every hour of every day.

**19.** A new lifter needs more protein than a weight-room veteran.

**20.** The older you are, the more protein you need.

**21.** Everything works better when you're strong.

**22.** There's no such thing as a fat-burning food.

**23.** All calories matter, whether they're going in or coming out.

# Notes

## Chapter 1. Membership Has Its Drawbacks

*How many people lift:* Kind of a tricky question. The U.S. Census Bureau reports that 34.5 million Americans seven or older participated in "weightlifting" more than once in 2009. Of course that leaves a lot of wiggle room. What seven-year-old is in a gym lifting weights? And "more than once" is astoundingly vague. So I got the 21 percent figure from some older data in this study: Julia Chevan, "Demographic determinants of participation in strength training activities among U.S. adults." *Journal of Strength and Conditioning Research* 2008; 22(2): 553–558. That study was based on data from the National Health Interview Survey, conducted in 2003. Fun fact from the survey: 3.7 percent of Americans claim to lift weights seven times a week.

*Self-efficacy:* The first paragraph refers to this study: James Annesi, "Supported exercise improves controlled eating and weight though its effects on psychosocial factors: extending a systematic research program toward treatment development." *The Permanente Journal* 2012; 16(1): 7–18. The study involved a population of obese, sedentary adults, who were put on an exercise program that started with walking or riding a stationary bike (although they were encouraged to do any type of exercise they wanted). There's only so much extrapolate to readers of the NROL series, but I wanted to include it because I've been reading Dr. Annesi's studies for a decade, and occasionally corresponding with him, so my awareness of the importance of self-efficacy begins with his work.

I based most of the section on this study: Gilson et al., "An examination of athletes' self-efficacy and strength training effort during an entire offseason." *Journal of Strength and Conditioning Research* 2012; 26(2): 443–451. The subjects here were Division I athletes (all male, alas) in football, volleyball, soccer, and basketball, who were followed for an entire off-season. A very cool feature of the study is that the athletes' self-evaluation was compared to the strength coaches' perception of their effort. The two measures tracked well, indicating that the athletes graded themselves honestly, perhaps because they knew their coaches would provide a reality check if they didn't.

*Reaching full potential: Designing Resistance Training Programs*, third edition, by Steven Fleck and William Kraemer (Human Kinetics, 2004). The information mostly comes from Chapter 2, "Types of Strength Training," pp. 13–51, although some comes from the following chapter, "Neuromuscular Physiology and Adaptations to Resistance Training."

## Chapter 2. The Six Movements You Need to Master

*Squat problems: Athletic Body in Balance*, by Gray Cook (Human Kinetics, 2003), p. 40.

*Fun facts about squats:* Clark et al., "Muscle activation in the loaded free barbell squat: a brief review." *Journal of Strength and Conditioning Research* 2012; 26(4): 1169–1178.

*Muscle trivia: The Book of Muscle*, by Ian King and Lou Schuler (Rodale, 2003).

*History of bench press:* Several years back I downloaded a lot of information from a site called americanpowerliftevolution.net. Alas, the site appears to be dead.

*Joe Weider vs. Bob Hoffman: Muscletown USA: Bob Hoffman and the Manly Culture of York Barbell*, by John D. Fair (Pennsylvania State University Press, 1999). It's one of my favorite reference books for information about the history of America's strength culture.

## Chapter 3. All Fitness Is Muscular Fitness

*Three components of fitness: Personal Trainer Manual* (American Council on Exercise, 1996).

*Dewey Cox:* He's the character played by John C. Reilly in *Walk Hard: The Dewey Cox Story*, which came out in 2007.

*Sitting:* James Vlahos, "Is Sitting a Lethal Activity?" *New York Times Magazine*, April 14, 2011.

*Strength and longevity:* See *The New Rules of Lifting*, page 5, and *The New Rules of Lifting for Women*, p. 12.

*Strength and performance:* McGuigan et al., "Strength training for athletes: does it really help sports performance?" *International Journal of Sports Physiology and Performance* 2012; 7: 2–5.

*Balance and performance:* Con Hrysomallis, "Balance ability and athletic performance." *Sports Medicine* 2011; 41(3): 221–232.

*Power training for athletes:* Cormie et al., "Adaptations in athletic performance after ballistic power versus strength training." *Medicine & Science in Sports & Exercise* 2010; 42(8): 1582–1598. I should mention that one of the coauthors is Rob Newton of Edith Cowan University in Australia. Dr. Newton's research in the 1990s and 2000s, starting when he was at Ball State University, broke new ground in the study of power performance. I quote him in Chapter 15.

*Power outage:* Reid and Fielding, "Skeletal muscle power: a critical determinant of physical functioning in older adults." *Exercise and Sports Sciences Reviews* 2012; 40(1): 4–12.

## Chapter 4. Bigger Is Better

*Hypertrophy mechanisms:* Brad Schoenfeld, "The mechanisms of muscle hypertrophy and their application to resistance training." *Journal of Strength and Conditioning Research* 2010; 24(10): 2857–2872. Brad Schoenfeld, "The Use of Specialized Training Techniques to Maximize Muscle Hypertrophy." *Strength and Conditioning Journal,* August 2011, pp. 60–65. I use these two papers throughout Chapter 4.

*Satellite cells:* Petrella et al., "Potent myofiber hypertrophy during resistance training in humans is associated with satellite cell-mediated myonuclear addition: a cluster analysis." *Journal of Applied Physiology* 2008; 104: 1736–1742.

*Load doesn't matter:* Mitchell et al., "Resistance exercise load does not determine training-mediated hypertrophic gains in young men." *Journal of Applied Physiology* 2012; 113(1): 71–77. I also referred to "How to Build Muscle with High Reps," by Christian Finn (muscleevo.net/how-to-build-muscle-with-high-reps/).

*Percentages of one-rep max: Essentials of Strength Training and Conditioning,* second edition (Human Kinetics, 2000), p. 407.

*Selecting inappropriate weights:* Ratamess et al., "Self-selected resistance training intensity in healthy women: the influence of a personal trainer." *Journal of Strength and Conditioning Research* 2008; 22(1): 103–111. Glass, "Effect of a learning trial on self-selected resistance training load." *Journal of Strength and Conditioning Research* 2008; 22(3): 1025–1029.

*Milo of Croton:* The basic story comes from Wikipedia (as does the note about the size of an adult bull's testicles). The calorie values are rough calculations from *Nutrition Almanac,* sixth edition, by John D. Kirschmann and Nutrition Search Inc. (McGraw-Hill, 2007). Michael Phelps's refutation that he or anyone else eats 12,000 calories a day was from an article on usatoday.com, dated May 10, 2012. Cattle birth and growth rates are from "Beef Cattle Breeds and Biological Types," by Scott P. Greiner, published by Virginia Cooperative Extension at Virginia Tech University.

*Strength and size gains:* This is from the second Schoenfeld article.

*Time under tension:* Most of this information came from the two Schoenfeld articles, along with this one: Scott, "The effect of time under tension and weight lifting cadence on aerobic, anaerobic, and recovery energy expenditures: three submaximal sets." *Applied Physiology, Nutrition, and Metabolism* 2012; 37(2): 252–256.

*Hypoxia:* This is from the first Schoenfeld citation.

## Chapter 5. The Care and Feeding of Your Muscles

*Alan Aragon and protein timing:* In *NROL for Life* (pp. 216–217) I credited Alan for changing my view on timing. Now I have to thank him again for helping me with *Supercharged*. With both books, Alan's presentations at the annual Fitness Summit in Kansas City (thefitnesssummit. com) led me to research I wouldn't otherwise have known about.

*Protein response in experienced vs. inexperienced lifters: Dietary Protein and Resistance Exercise (DPRE)*, edited by Lonnie Lowery and Jose Antonio (CRC Press, 2012), pp. 84–87. The quote from Stuart Phillips came via e-mail in response to a question I asked about this area of research.

*Misinformation about health risks of dietary protein: DPRE*, pp. 41–68. Lonnie Lowery, a nutrition professor at Winona State University and one of the book's editors (also a friend and longtime source of cutting-edge information), uses this chapter to thoroughly debunk every anti-protein trope you've come across, and probably a few you haven't.

*Protein and older lifters:* Yang et al., "Resistance exercise enhances myofibrillar protein synthesis with graded intakes of whey protein in older men." *British Journal of Nutrition* 2012; Feb 7:1–9 (epub ahead of print). Once again, I have to credit Alan Aragon for the heads-up on this study. Also *DPRE*, pp. 158–159.

*Women vs. men: DPRE*, pp. 136–139.

*Muscle breakdown/post-workout protein synthesis rate:* Churchward-Venne et al., "Nutritional regulation of muscle protein synthesis with resistance exercise: strategies to enhance anabolism." *Nutrition and Metabolism* 2012; May 17; 9(1): 40 (epub ahead of print).

*Mike Roussell:* Mike is a friend and occasional collaborator. You can check out his work at mikeroussell.com. He used the light-switch analogy in his "Ask the Macro Manager" Q-and-A column at bodybuilding.com, posted June 22, 2012.

*Leucine required to maximize protein synthesis: DPRE*, pages 84–85.

*Leucine in common foods: Nutrition Almanac*, sixth edition, by John D. Kirschmann and Nutrition Search Inc. (McGraw-Hill, 2007).

*Liquid meal replacements:* Conley et al., "Effect of food form on postprandial amino acid concentrations in older adults." *British Journal of Nutrition* 2011; 106(2): 203–207.

*Whey vs. casein vs. soy: DPRE,* pp. 102–111. Also Churchward-Venne et al., previously cited.

*Creatine: DPRE,* pp. 178–188.

## Chapter 6. Let's Get Small

*Vince Gironda and pre-steroid-era nutrition:* "Remembering the Guru: Vince Gironda, the Greatest Trainer Who Ever Lived," by Ron Kosloff (criticalbench.com/VinceGironda.htm).

*Crap foods: NROL for Abs,* pp. 195–201, and *NROL for Life,* pp. 227–235.

*Paleo diet article:* The article ran in the October 2012 issue of *Men's Health.*

*Paleo diet history:* Marlene Zuk, "The Evolutionary Search for Our Perfect Past." *New York Times,* January 19, 2009.

*Weight-loss maintenance:* Ebbeling et al., "Effects of dietary composition on energy expenditure during weight-loss maintenance." *Journal of the American Medical Association* 2012; 307(24): 2627–2634.

*Substrate metabolism:* Galgani and Ravussin, "Energy metabolism, fuel selection, and body-weight regulation." *International Journal of Obesity* 2008; 32 (supplement 7): S109–S119. Hopkins et al., "The relationship between substrate metabolism, exercise, and appetite control." *Sports Medicine* 2011; 41(6): 507–521.

*A million calories a year:* This assumes the 150-pounder is eating 2,750 calories a day, which would be low for an athlete and probably high for a woman trying to shave a few pounds of fat from that starting weight. But, with apologies, I wanted to use some nice round numbers, even if they don't quite work together.

## Chapter 8. Squat

*Muscles used in squat:* I may not have written that exact sentence, but if you combine two sentences in *The Book of Muscle* (pp. 2 and 198), you get pretty close. Thomas Myers is author of *Anatomy Trains* (Churchill Livingstone, 2001). I got the "one muscle, 600 compartments" idea from his presentation at the Perform Better Functional Training Summit in June 2011 in Providence, Rhode Island. I didn't write fast enough to get his exact quote, but what I have is pretty close.

*Front squat:* Stephen P. Bird and Sean Casey, "Exploring the Front Squat." *Strength and Conditioning Journal,* April 2012, pp. 27–33. See also *Starting Strength,* third edition, by Mark Rippetoe (The Aasgaard Company, 2011), pp. 243–249.

*Back squat and sports: Essentials of Strength Training and Conditioning,* second edition, p. 309.

*Trap-bar deadlift:* For a good discussion of how the trap-bar deadlift compares with conventional and sumo deadlifts, see "Deadlifts: Which Type Is Best for You?" by Mike Robertson, t-nation.com, April 25, 2012. To read more about how the line blurs between squats and deadlifts, see "Deadlift or Squat: What's the Diff?" by Michael Boyle, also at t-nation.com, May 2, 2012. Boyle says that the only clear difference between the two exercises is that the weight is on your shoulders with a squat and in your hands with a deadlift. (Although he points out that this only applies to bilateral barbell exercises; when you use dumbbells on lunges or single-leg-stance exercises the definitions blur even more.)

## Chapter 9. Hinge

*Conventional vs. trap-bar deadlift:* Swinton et al., "A biomechanical analysis of straight and hexagonal barbell deadlifts using submaximal loads." *Journal of Strength and Conditioning Research* 2011; 25(7): 2000–2009.

## Chapter 10. Push

*Dumbbell fly:* Welsch et al., "Electromyographic activity of the pectoralis major and anterior deltoid muscles during three upper-body lifts." *Journal of Strength and Conditioning Research* 2005; 19(2): 449–452.

*Bench press angles:* Trebs et al., "An electromyography analysis of three muscles surrounding the shoulder joint during performance of a chest press exercise at several angles." *Journal of Strength and Conditioning Research* 2010; 24(7): 1925–1930.

## Chapter 11. Pull

*Heavy shrugs: Starting Strength*, p. 236.

## Chapter 14. Core Training

*Sit-up test:* I got the test from "How Strong Are Your Abs, Really?," an article written by my friend Nick Tumminello, which was posted on t-nation.com on January 26, 2009. (I edited the article; it was one of my favorites.)

*Spinal rotation: Low Back Disorders,* by Stuart McGill, Ph.D. (Human Kinetics, 2002), p. 88.

*Role of hip flexors:* This comes from two different sources: McGill's *Low Back Disorders,* pp. 72–74 and 104–108, and Thomas Myers's *Anatomy Trains* (Churchill Livingstone, 2001), Chapter 9.

## Chapter 15. Combination and Power Exercises

*Jump squat quote:* The quote from Dr. Newton is from an e-mail, as noted in the text.

*Explosive push-up pros and cons:* Garcia-Masso et al., "Myoelectric activation and kinetics of different plyometric push-up variations." *Journal of Strength and Conditioning Research* 2011; 25(7): 2040–2047.

## Chapter 17. RAMP It Up, Tone It Down

*Effects of adrenaline on workout: Essentials of Strength Training and Conditioning*, p. 112.

## Chapter 21. Strength & Power

*Powerlifting contest:* Rachel Cosgrove deadlifted 297 pounds in a USA Powerlifting California State Championship on March 1, 2008. She competed in the women's "raw" division, which means without special powerlifting equipment beyond a belt.

# Index

*Page numbers in italics refer to illustrations.*